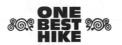
ONE
BEST
HIKE

YOSEMITE'S
HALF DOME

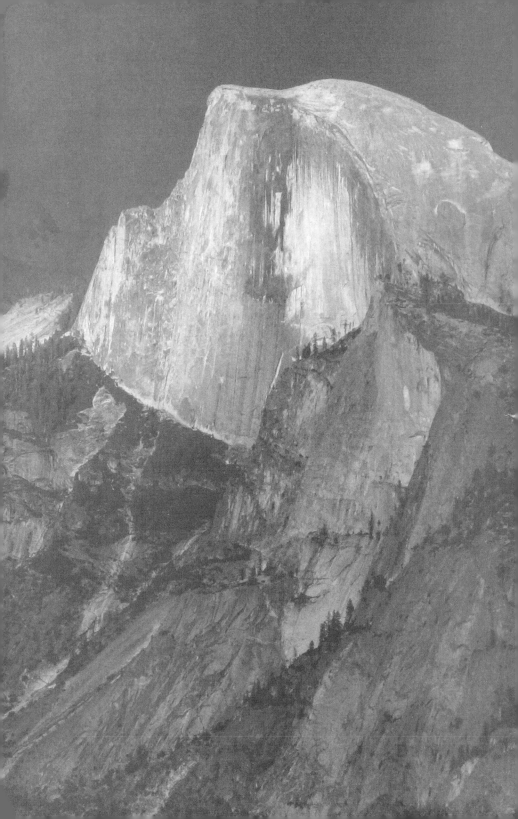

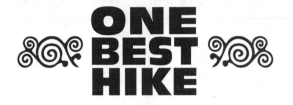

ONE
BEST
HIKE

YOSEMITE'S HALF DOME

Everything you need to know to successfully hike Yosemite's most famous landmark

SECOND EDITION

Rick Deutsch

 WILDERNESS PRESS ... *on the trail since 1967*

One Best Hike: Yosemite's Half Dome

2nd EDITION 2012

Text and photos by the author, except where indicated.
Cover design: Larry B. Van Dyke and Scott McGrew
Book design and layout: Andreas Schueller and Annie Long

Library of Congress Cataloging-in-Publication Data

Deutsch, Rick.
    One best hike : Yosemite's Half Dome / Rick Deutsch. — 2nd ed.
    p. cm.
    Includes bibliographical references and index.
    ISBN-13: 978-0-89997-674-7
    ISBN-10: 0-89997-674-3
    1. Hiking—California—Yosemite National Park—Guidebooks.
    2. Hiking—California—Half Dome—Guidebooks. 3. Half Dome
    (Calif.)—Guidebooks. 4. Yosemite National Park (Calif.)—Guidebooks. I. Title.
    GV199.42.C22Y664 2012
    917.94'47—dc23
                                2011053068
Manufactured in the United States of America

Published by: **Wilderness Press**
                  P.O. Box 43673
                  Birmingham, Alabama 35243
                  info@wildernesspress.com
                  www.wildernesspress.com
Visit our website for a complete list of our books and for ordering information.

Distributed by Publishers Group West

SAFETY NOTICE: Although Wilderness Press and the author have made every attempt to ensure that the information in this book is accurate at press time, they are not responsible for any loss, damage, injury, or inconvenience that may occur to anyone while using this book. Readers are advised to recheck phone numbers, prices, addresses, and other material. You are responsible for your own safety and health while in the wilderness. The fact that a trail is described in this book does not mean that it will be safe for you. The potential for falls, heat exhaustion, dehydration, hyperventilation, or other problems are possible (though not likely). Be aware that trail conditions can change from day to day. Always check local conditions and the weather, and know your own limitations.

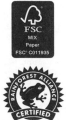

Acknowledgments

I would like to thank:

My wife, Diane, for her patience during my many hikes of Half Dome, my training, and the hours I spent at the keyboard.

My sister, Michelle Deutsch LaMarche, who did the hike before me and encouraged me to do it the first time.

The National Park Service and the Yosemite Conservancy for their support of this precious American resource.

Dan Anderson for his efforts in digitizing many of the early Yosemite historical manuscripts in the Yosemite Online Library so that everyone may enjoy them.

Harv Galic for his compilation of the *Chronicles of Early Ascents of Half Dome.*

The many new friendships that Half Dome has introduced me to, including Sonke Kastner, Sister Kathy Littrell, Scott Gehrman, Pat Townsley, NPS ranger Mark Marschall, NPS ranger Daniel Schaible, Pete Devine (Yosemite Conservancy), and my many Facebook fans, blog readers, and audiences.

My hiking buddy, Yosey (as in Yosemite), a 5-pound Yorkie whose zest for life inspires me.

Rick Deutsch
Mr. Half Dome

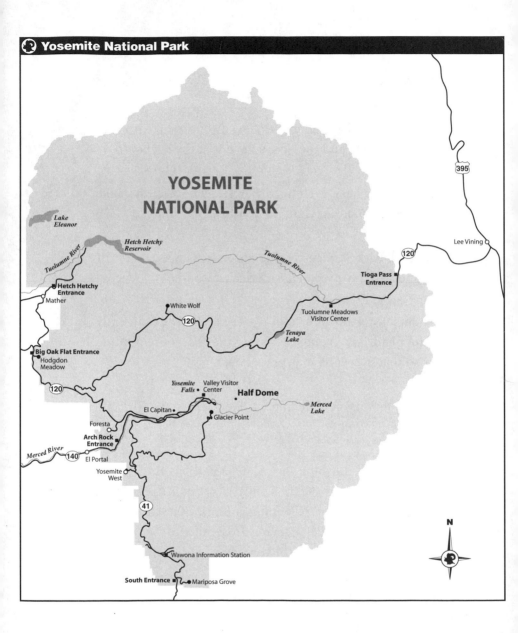

YOSEMITE
NATIONAL PARK

Lake Eleanor

Hetch Hetchy Reservoir

Lee Vining

Tuolumne River

Tuolumne River

395

120

Tioga Pass Entrance

Hetch Hetchy Entrance

Mather

White Wolf

120

Tuolumne Meadows Visitor Center

Big Oak Flat Entrance

Hodgdon Meadow

Tenaya Lake

120

Yosemite Falls

Valley Visitor Center

Half Dome

El Capitan

Merced Lake

Foresta

Glacier Point

Arch Rock Entrance

Merced River

140

El Portal

Yosemite West

41

N

Wawona Information Station

South Entrance

Mariposa Grove

Contents

Foreword

I heartily recommend this book. It is a well-written and thorough guide to reaching the top of my favorite Yosemite rock form. Why is Half Dome my favorite? Because it stands alone at the east end of Yosemite Valley. It isn't as big as El Capitan, 7 miles to the west. With its 3,000-foot south face, El Capitan guards the gates of the valley. But Half Dome has a 2,000-foot northwest face that is straight up and down, a summit that isn't reachable by merely hiking a trail through the forest, and the Dome is almost 2,000 feet higher than El Cap. Half Dome was first climbed in 1875 by George Anderson, a Scot (John Muir, another Scot, reached the summit of Cathedral Peak in 1869). These days Half Dome is ascended tens of thousands of times a year. Why? Because people want to be able to say, as they look up from the valley, "I've been there." Once, the author of this book, after complimenting me on having made the first ascent of the great face of Half Dome, claimed that "Of course, I went up the easy way." As I said to Rick then and say to you, dear reader, now, "There's no easy way up Half Dome." Getting to the top requires a nearly 16-mile round-trip and an elevation gain of almost 5,000 feet. That's a bit of work for a day, but you can do it. I would read carefully what Rick Deutsch has to say in this revised second edition, especially about being fit. You want to be fit and to have good footwear.

Rick has had to revise this guide to hiking Half Dome. Things change, and the guide has to change with them. In particular, there is now a permit system to ascend the cable stairway of Half Dome. Yes, I know, permit systems are a bother. Oh, for the days when we could spend the night on top of Half Dome. The park service instituted the permit system to cut down on the crowding that was occurring on the cables. There have been a few serious accidents that were attributable to so many people being up there at the same time. Rick now includes a thorough guide to navigating the permit system.

The only place where I differ significantly from Rick is on starting time. Rick recommends an early start. I agree. But where Rick suggests 6 a.m., I am for 3 a.m. I know it is hard to get up that early, but if you do you will never be sorry. You will hike up in the cool of the morning and reach the top ahead of the crowds, so much ahead of them that you will be able to descend the cables before they arrive and start up. Rick also says that June is his favorite time of year in Yosemite. I prefer the fall. It's true that the waterfalls have dried up, but there are no bugs, the air is clear, the Mist Trail is dry, and the people have left.

Have a good hike and remember, you are going to the best summit in the Yosemite region.

Royal Robbins
Modesto, CA
March 2012

Note: Royal Robbins led the first group to climb the 1,800-foot-high Regular Northwest Face route on Half Dome in 1957.

Preface

The motto for my life is "carpe diem." This is a Latin phrase meaning "seize the day." It is believed to have originated with the ancient philosopher Horace, the leading Roman lyric poet during the time of Augustus Caesar. The phrase was made popular in the 1989 movie *Dead Poets Society,* starring Robin Williams. He invoked his students: "Carpe diem! Seize the day, lads. Make your lives extraordinary!" Another interpretation would be: "Smell the rose today, for it may be wilted tomorrow."

My first Half Dome hike, in 1990, was a life-changing experience. It was so much fun and so challenging that I decided to do it every year. It made me realize that if I was to experience all life had to offer, I had to get planning. I wrote a life list (now called a bucket list, a term made popular by the 2007 film starring Jack Nicholson and Morgan Freeman) to make sure I did the things I wanted to do. Prior to Half Dome I said, "Someday I want to see the pyramids; someday I will see the Taj Mahal; someday I will walk on the Great Wall." When you are young, you have a lot of "somedays." But in reality, someday often never comes. I have carried my life list for more than 20 years and checked off many things. For me it's a living list—I constantly add things. I had never heard of Jordan's treasure, Petra, five years ago and now I've been there. Looking back, for me Half Dome was the start of this awareness. We all have a finite number of heartbeats allocated to us, and one day tomorrow will not come. Our personal life odometer clicks over relentlessly; too soon you're 30, 40, 50, and beyond. It seems to spin too fast. What you do with your time is your decision. You have a choice: Sit on the sidelines and watch the world on your TV or get out and live life. Experience things while you can; hike Half Dome.

Try this exercise. Write down all the things you want to do or see or experience before you die. Now write down the number of years you think you will remain ambulatory and able to physically and mentally attempt those things. Next, consider how much free time you will have available. This should be your private list—only put down the things that you personally want to do. And remember that you'll likely use some of your vacation time for weddings, funerals, and family events. A few of your major wants may take two weeks or more (a safari, a trip to Antarctica, a bike ride across America). You will see that there is not enough time left to do the whole list—let alone repeat the spectacular ones. Put down the TV remote and strap on your hiking boots, ride your bike, swim, run, or just smell that rose today.

In this second edition, I have incorporated a wealth of learning gained about Half Dome and the early days of Yosemite. I expanded on much of the early Yosemite history and geology and added GPS points to help you arrive at the points of interest. At press time I had done the hike 31 times. Half Dome is my passion; make it yours.

I'll do my best to get you to the top of your mountain. You *can* do Half Dome with three things: education, preparation, and motivation. I will help teach you what you need to know. You have to do the prep work. Hike a lot of hills and build up your upper body strength for the pull up the famous cables. Do the hike because *you* want to do it. What is your motivation? Half Dome is a goal and a journey. Have fun!

Carpe diem!
Rick Deutsch "Mr. Half Dome"
www.HikeHalfDome.com

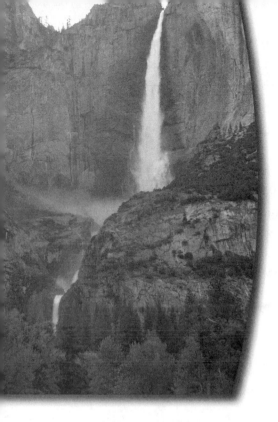

Introduction

No temple made with hands can compare with Yosemite. Every rock in its walls seems to glow with life . . . . The true ownership of the wilderness belongs in the highest to those who love it most.

—John Muir

Yosemite—the very name evokes images of verdant valleys, cascading waterfalls, peaceful meadows, soaring mountains, arching domes, meandering rivers, lush forests, diverse wildlife, and 2,000-year-old giant sequoias. These 1,200 square miles, located in Northern California's Sierra Nevada mountain range, are the crown jewel of the National Park Service. Yosemite has become a must-see on the list of every outdoor enthusiast. The park's natural wonders attract people of all kinds, be they old, young, citizens, or foreigners. Nearly 4 million people come each year. With this popularity comes the crush of humanity—out to explore the wonders of nature, many sporting only a backpack, a bottle of water, and a desire to see nature as it has existed for centuries. Yosemite's hikes are superb, from short jaunts to expeditions of several days. The Yosemite Valley comprises only 1% of the park but is the most popular destination in this paradise; 95% of Yosemite is designated wilderness.

In the wilderness we can seek solitude, devoid of human impact. Recognize that being in the wilderness brings responsibility. You must assess any risks you may encounter and deal with them appropriately. Hiking, climbing, bouldering, encountering wildlife, and gazing over cliffs can be risky. This includes the exhilarating trek up Half Dome. No one will tell you that you cannot go up. No one is there to log you in, examine your gear, or make a judgment as to your ability to do this hike. Beyond the park-wide regulations guiding safety and resource protection, prohibiting certain activities such as BASE jumping, there are only two specific official rules: (1) You cannot camp above 7,900 feet (including the summit), and (2) you need a permit to be on Sub Dome and the cables (more on this in Chapter 7, Preparation).

The Yosemite General Management Plan, drawn up in 1980, cites as one of its goals the promotion of visitor understanding and enjoyment. This is in direct support of the 1864 original Yosemite Grant, signed by President Abraham Lincoln in the midst of the Civil War. The Yosemite Valley and the Mariposa Grove of Big Trees were the first public lands set aside for the people. The 1890 designation as a national park ensured that Yosemite would be available to citizens for their enjoyment, education, and recreation, now and in the future. This book, *One Best Hike: Yosemite's Half Dome*, serves as a vehicle to help achieve this goal.

In a great honor, Yosemite was selected as the theme for California on the 2005 U.S. quarter. California's quarter depicts naturalist and conservationist John Muir admiring a condor and Yosemite's monolithic granite headwall known as Half Dome. It bears the inscriptions "California," "John

Muir," "Yosemite Valley," and "1850," the year the state was admitted to the Union. Yosemite was honored on the quarter again in 2010, with 3,000-foot-high El Capitan featured. When you consider the varied attractions in California, 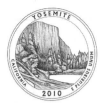 it is indeed a testament to have Yosemite represent the Golden State to the country and the world. Yosemite has been recognized internationally as well: in 1984 it was designated a World Heritage Site by the United Nations.

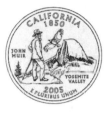

Yosemite's rugged backcountry and 800 miles of trails afford plenty of opportunity to discover oneself. Of all the hikes possible in the park, one of the most popular day hikes is to the top of the signature landmark of the park, Half Dome. Located at the eastern edge of Yosemite Valley, Half Dome is the most hiked mountains in the Sierra Nevada, with more than 40,000 ascents per year. This is a big hike—a full 10- to 12-hour day for most people, comprising nearly 16 miles round-trip. Add to this the 4,737-foot vertical rise (and fall) and the Half Dome hike becomes an extremely strenuous one. Included is a harrowing 425-foot vertical climb up the approximately 45-degree incline of the back side of the granite slope. Not to worry; this is accomplished with the aid of two steel cable handrails.

This guide is for everyone—the person who is not toting the latest in GPS gear or topographical maps of all the nooks and crannies of the park. It's for those who have a genuine interest in learning about the history of the park, the lives of the Native Americans, and the geology that created these formations, as well as the roles of early explorers and modern conservationists. The focus is on Half Dome. It's for the person who has thought about doing the hike but doesn't know much about it. I believe that anyone can successfully complete this hike with three things: education, preparation, and motivation. This book, my website, my blog, my talks, my free Web-enabled device app, and other resources will help with your education. Preparation is up to you. Take this hike seriously. Walking your dog a mile a night will not get you into condition. Your training hikes need to include many hills. If you live in an area without vertical challenges, climb up and down the fire escape stairs in a local high-rise. Finally, be motivated for *your* reasons and don't be dragged along by friends if this effort is beyond your capability. The hike is both a goal and a journey. Your adventure will involve strength, risk, and discovery, and this guide will prepare you to be self-reliant.

The hike can be done in one day, or more leisurely in two if time permits. This guidebook describes the most popular day route to the summit. Regardless of your strategy, it will help you prepare prior to leaving home and then help steer you up the mountain on your summit day. My intent is to provide a resource that can enable nearly any physically able person to complete the hike. Further, I believe that this educational guide will enhance visitor understanding and enjoyment of park resources.

I first hiked Half Dome in 1990 and was so moved by the experience that I decided to do it annually. My motivation goes back to the sixth-century tale of Milo of Croton (it was a Greek colony in southern Italy). As a boy, Milo would pick up a small calf on a daily basis. As the calf grew larger, Milo continued to lift the animal, and the boy became stronger. His muscles became so powerful that he could carry the calf with ease when it became a full-size ox. This constant yet gradual training resulted in Milo developing into a man of incredible strength, so much so that he won the ancient Olympic wrestling title a remarkable six consecutive times. He was likely an actual historical person, as he is mentioned by many classical authors, among them Aristotle. Perhaps this is a poor analogy, but maybe by working out on a regular basis and staying in condition for this hike, I will live a few years longer than the actuarial tables project.

While on these hikes, I have noticed many unprepared optimists setting out, knowing little of what lies ahead. Their poor preparation was obvious. I have seen many people suffer from a lack of water, sore muscles, inferior shoes, and a big underestimation of the magnitude of the hike. And yet, I've found no other Half Dome–specific hiking guides. You'll find many general hiking in Yosemite guidebooks, but they cover Half Dome in only a few pages. This guide should fill your knowledge gaps and allow you to hit the trail with confidence.

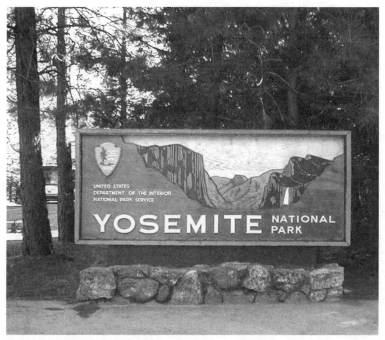

Welcome to Yosemite!

This book was designed to be small and fit into your pack, so take it on your hike. Many people will be on the trail—you won't get lost. I've included photos of most of the trail, so you won't wonder what's in store. Although these pictures show the high points of the hike, nothing will replace seeing these majestic sights yourself. I also include many historical vignettes of events that occurred during the evolution of Yosemite. Finally, all opinions and suggestions are mine. Others may approach these topics differently or disagree with me. Pick out what you like and make informed decisions.

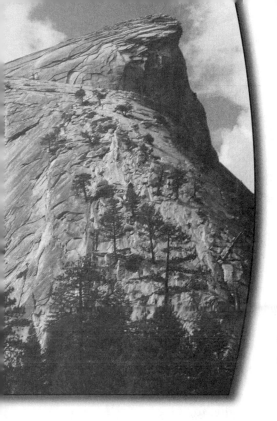

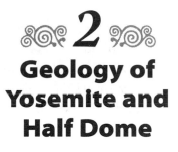

❦ *2* ❦
Geology of Yosemite and Half Dome

When we try to pick out anything by itself, we find it hitched to everything else in the Universe.

—John Muir

How Yosemite Was Formed

Yosemite's grandeur began about 500 million years ago, when the entire region was an ancient seabed. Since the beginning, the plates that make up the outer portion of the Earth have been moving—coming together and breaking apart. Witness how nicely eastern South America fits into western Africa. About 100 million years ago, the plate west of today's California, called the Pacific plate, dove eastward under the North American plate, causing the uplift of the region. The mountains still rise today at a rate of 1 foot every 1,000 years. Deep below the ground, constant Earth movement and the effects of pressure and heat created magma, which gradually rose toward the surface. When the magma found boundaries or rifts between the surface plates (subduction zones), it rose up to erupt as volcanoes. This is a phenomenon that happens regularly on Earth. However, sometimes the hot 2,000-degree magma has no route to the surface. It rises but then is forced to lie a few miles below the surface and slowly cool under intense pressure. It then crystallizes into a pluton of granite. When many of these plutons come together, they become batholiths. There are many types of granite, but most consist of a chemical mixture of hornblende, mica, feldspar, quartz, and other minerals. Its classic look is a salt-and-pepper gray, but the color can vary. It can have different patterns and lines due to intrusions during its formation.

In California, as the Pacific plate slowly crawled under the North American plate, the subduction zone got extremely hot and melted some of the plate, along with some of the overlying crust. Because of the temperature difference with the rocks around it, the magma rose and formed the Sierra granite directly from this subducting slab. This huge mass would later become the underlay of the Sierra Nevada mountains. Most of Yosemite's granites were formed 85–150 million years ago. Add to the recipe the millions of years of erosion caused by snow, rain, and wind, and gradually the batholiths were exposed. One result was the 80-by-400-mile granite bedrock of the Sierra Nevada.

The best reader-friendly book on Yosemite's formation is *Geology Underfoot in Yosemite National Park*. It was cowritten by Allen F. Glazner, professor of geological sciences at the University of North Carolina, and ranger Greg Stock, the first-ever park geologist at Yosemite. The advances in technology, such as optical remote sensing, high-resolution photography, seismic monitoring, and rockfall runout simulations, are now part of the park's tools to study rockfalls.

From about 10–3 million
years ago, the Merced and
Tuolumne rivers carved
down deep into the land
with greater intensity. The
uplifted land gave more
gravitational power to the
river. The eroded earth
gradually found its way
into the Central Valley.

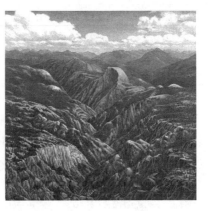

Uplift and river erosion

Then, from about 3 million to 18,000 years ago, global cooling resulted in three major glacial periods. Glaciers are simply
large masses of snow and ice that do not melt. The snow and
ice filled in valleys and accumulated thousands of feet high.
Gravity allowed them to slowly advance. As the lower layer of
ice picked up rocks, it carved the path of the glacier. The repre-
sentation below reflects geologists' belief that Half Dome and
many other high peaks were above the glaciers. We will discuss
the geologic formation of Half Dome in the next section.

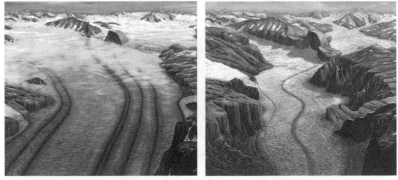

Early glaciation   Recent glaciation

The last major glacier retreated from Yosemite about 18,000
years ago. (We still have two glaciers: Mount Lyell and Mount
Maclure.) The classic U shape of glacially carved valleys is not

All illustrations this page and next by Eric Knight (Modified from Matthes, 1939);
courtesy of the National Park Service

readily evident in Yosemite Valley because research has shown that the bedrock lies about 2,000 feet below today's roads. How did that happen? During its time, the last glacier slowly covered the area between El Capitan and Bridalveil Fall. As it dug deep, stone and debris were deposited in front of it. When it finally melted and retreated back to the east, the terminal moraine created an earthen dam. The dam stopped the waters from the melting ice and created a lake that geologists call Yosemite Lake. By 10,000 years ago, the lake had filled with sediment, disguising the U shape. Scientists believe the U shape is still there—it's just 2,000 feet below the surface.

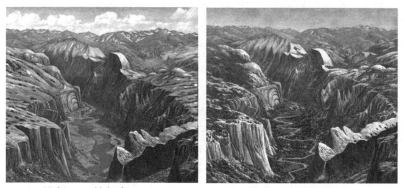

Melting and lake formation   Present day Yosemite

Yosemite is undergoing change even today. Being relatively young geologically, the area is still settling in. Earthquakes have been reported since records were kept in the mid-1800s. Rockfalls are very common at Yosemite. Since 1857, more than 500 rockfalls in Yosemite Valley have killed 14 people and injured more than 60, more than at any other national park. They are the result of quakes and a process of exfoliation, that is, large sheets of granite peeling off in vertical patterns similar to an onion skin. Rockfalls also occur when rainwater gets into cracks and freezes. When water freezes, it expands. The small but constant expansion may cause the granite to open slightly. Lichens can grow here, and when they die, they provide a soil structure in which larger plants can germinate. In time, the growing plant exerts forces that can lead to a flaking off. Given enough time, these processes can take their toll.

In the 1980s a major rockfall occurred off the Three Brothers formation. In 1996 and again in 1999, enormous sheets of granite dropped near Happy Isles; each event killed one person. The impact produced massive shock waves that literally snapped thousands of trees. The 1996 rockfall was comprised of two slabs (totaling 80,000 tons) bigger than two football fields and three stories tall. They free-fell 1,800 feet and had reached a velocity of 270 miles per hour when they impacted. In 2008 a rockfall off the Glacier Point wall behind Curry Village took more than 200 tent cabins and wooden cabins out of service. You can still see the talus fields from this fall. In 2009 a rockfall even larger than the 1996 Happy Isles fall occurred at Ahwiyah Point near the eastern side of Half Dome's face. An estimated 115 tons of rock crashed down onto the southern portion of the Mirror Lake Loop Trail. When you are on top of Half Dome, you can carefully crawl out to the edge and look down at the fresh white stone talus field at Ahwiyah Point.

Flooding has also changed the landscape of the park. The Merced River flood of 1997 set records, and the high water marks are still visible. It caused $178 million in damage in Yosemite Valley. As a result, the valley was closed for more than three months, and vast changes were made to the area's management plan. Today numerous structures have been relocated, roads have been rerouted out of the flood plain, and nearly 50% of campsites have been removed.

In 2006 spring rains created a huge rockslide southwest of El Portal that dropped tons of earth from Ferguson Ridge onto CA 140, closing that road for part of the year. Today travel is only possible via two one-way Bailey bridges, which take traffic

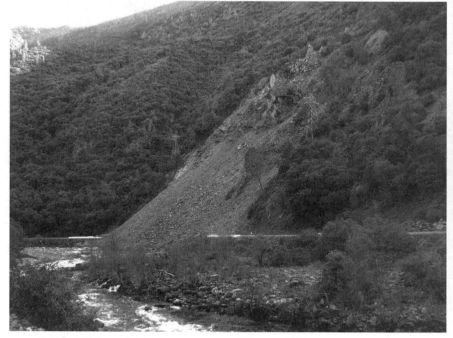

Ferguson Ridge rockslide

across the Merced and onto the remnants of the old Yosemite Railroad track, then back 0.25 mile later. The train ceased operation in 1945, and the track was sold off for scrap.

Occasional fires ravage parts of the park with the loss of thousands of acres of forest. Lightning is most often the cause, but man-made fires also take their toll. An out-of-control prescribed burn in August 2009 in the Big Meadow area near Foresta devastated nearly 8,000 acres. These unpredictable phenomena are reminders of Yosemite's dynamic state.

How Half Dome Was Formed

Half Dome is estimated to be nearly 90 million years old. It is the signature landmark of Yosemite and is truly an American and a global icon. (It was the inspiration for the logo of the North Face company.) It is one of the planet's most vertical walls, with the face rising 2,000 feet straight up. Its peak reaches an altitude of 8,842 feet. The distinctive face reflects Earth's primordial power. Unlike most domes in the park, such as Liberty Cap, it is not a true spherical dome. When viewed from the west, it appears as a rounded table rather then the half-ball image it presents from other angles. It's estimated that only 20% of the original dome is gone.

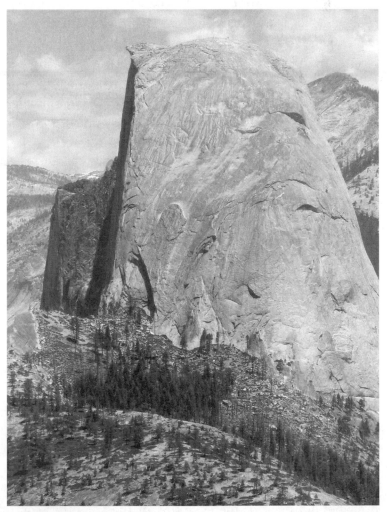

Only 20% "missing"

The exact method of Half Dome's formation is not totally understood. When I moved to California, I was told straightaway that it was cut in half by glaciers. That explanation makes sense, and it certainly looks that way, but that is mostly wrong. It is true that Half Dome's shape was influenced by glaciers; the northern and southern sides were affected about halfway up. Even John Muir believed it was glacial in origin. Yosemite likely has more granite domes than anywhere else on Earth, and most were indeed formed by glaciers. However, today's geologists feel certain that Half Dome stood above the glaciers, as did many of the higher peaks in the park. No classic striations are on its surface or upper slopes. Another telltale sign is the erratic that rests at the Diving Board (western edge of the face) at 7,500 feet. An erratic is a large boulder that the glacier carries along and then gently puts down as it retreats. This boulder has the same material as the Cathedral Peak granite and is not the same as the Half Dome granodiorite that makes up the Diving Board. Clearly, this erratic was deposited by a glacier at that point.

When viewed from the air or from Washburn or Glacier points, Half Dome appears as part of a ridge along Tenaya Canyon. Scientists call this ridge a vertically oriented joint. The internal compression pressure in the rock causes it to develop joint plates that align themselves with the surface, regardless of the slope of the surface.

Glaciers did carve the lower ends of Half Dome, up to about 700 feet from the top, resulting in overhangs. These overhangs were released by the exfoliation action of the joints over time. So, it is safe to say that we don't know definitively how Half Dome got its shape, but the face was probably caused by rockfalls and exfoliation along a prominent vertically oriented fracture on the famous north face, and glaciers probably did most of the sculpting of the smoother south face. Regardless, it is unique and beautiful.

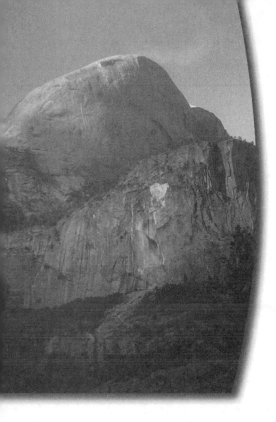

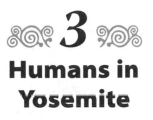

3

Humans in Yosemite

Climb the mountains and get their good tidings. Nature's peace will flow into you as sunshine flows into trees. The winds will blow their own freshness into you, and the storms their energy, while cares will drop off like autumn leaves.

—John Muir

Native Americans

The earliest Native Americans arrived in the area about 8,000 years ago. By the time of the European explorers, the Native American tribes in the greater California region included about 90 distinct entities. The Spanish were the dominant foreigners, and they focused their activities on religious conversion and raising cattle. The burgeoning Mexican territory meant they were spread thin in the west. The Native Americans living here were mostly agrarian and did not unify into a strong fighting machine, as did the Sioux, Cherokee, or Lakota of the plains. They did not rebel against the Spaniards. From 1769 to 1823, the Spaniards began a rigorous mission construction program, wherein each of 21 California missions was located about a day's walk from the next. The missions ranged from Mission San Diego de Alcalá in the south to Mission San Francisco Solano, in Sonoma, to the north. The goal of converting the locals consumed much of the daily life for the Spaniards, and they did not venture deep into the Sierra but instead built settlements in the coastal and central valley areas. In the mid-1800s some of the tribes in the Sierra area were the Po-ho-nee-chees, Po-to-en'-cies, Wil-tuc-um'-nees, Noot'-choos, Chow-chil'-las, Ho-na'-ches, Me'-woos, Monos, and the Chook-chan'-ces. Today some of these names live on at Native American casinos in the area.

The tribe that called Yosemite Valley home was related to the Miwok and Mono Paiute. They called themselves Ahwahneechee, which is believed to mean "place of the gaping mouth." (The entrance to the valley resembles such.)

Arrival of the Whites

By the early 1800s the American frontier of the time lay to the west of St. Joseph, Missouri. There were no towns or settlements to speak of farther west. The mountains of the High Sierra were unknown to the Anglos who were migrating westward. The exploratory journey of Meriwether Lewis

Today the National Park Service takes care to get the involvement of many tribes when they conduct projects that impact the park. Specifically, the following are consulted: American Indian Council of Mariposa County, Bishop Paiute Tribal Office, North Fork Mono Rancheria, Bridgeport Paiute Indian Colony, Picayune Rancheria of Chukchansi Indians, Mono Lake Kutzadika'a Paiute Tribe, and the Tuolumne Band of Me-Wuk Indians.

and William Clark provided the first organized route to the new western continent. Surprisingly, it was the East Coast and European fashion industry that helped drive western exploration. Furs had become the wrap of choice for society women in Boston, Philadelphia, New York, and Paris. The high price that soft beaver pelts could bring trappers spurred on an industry to seek the mammals. Trails penetrating the Rocky Mountains began to appear, and thousands of beavers and other fur-bearing animals lured rugged trappers onto uncharted lands. The players in this cottage industry would meet annually to trade their bounty for cash with resellers. Yearly meetings (not unlike the buyer-seller conventions of today) were called rendezvous. Trappers, guides, suppliers, and ambitious men would recruit hunting parties to venture into the unknown. Skilled Native Americans were allowed to participate in a gesture of equality. In July 1833 the rendezvous was held on the banks of the Green River in Utah. It was here that a man named Captain Joseph Walker assembled a fur-hunting party. His goal was to find a direct westward route for trappers through the Central Sierra to the Pacific Coast. (The first westward expedition to California was accomplished by Jedediah Smith in 1826, but that route was via the easier southern Sierra and into San Diego.) Historical research into the journals of one member of the Walker party, Zenas Leonard, allows us to reconstruct the Walker route with some confidence. It appears the men traveled west to Salt Lake, and then followed the Humboldt River into western Nevada and on to Mono Lake before attempting to cross the High Sierra. The expedition then passed by the East Fork of the Walker River and by areas we know today as Glen Aulin and Tenaya Lake. Of interest here is the very high probability that they actually continued on and looked down into Yosemite Valley from a vantage at Yosemite Point. Their descriptions appear to accurately reflect this. The party did not descend into the valley but continued on their quest through Crane Flat, Merced Grove, and then along the lower Merced into San Francisco, Gilroy, and finally Monterey. Extensive research, including hiking these trails, by authors Grant Hiskes and John Hiskes (*The Discovery of Yosemite 1833*) helped confirm these facts.

A few others are thought to be the first to see Yosemite Valley. One could have been James Savage. He ran trading posts in the region, managed to marry five Native American women, and spoke their language. When both his Fresno River and South Fork trading posts were raided by Native Americans and some deaths resulted, it is highly probable that he pursued the renegades up the Merced River Valley and eventually into Yosemite Valley. Other candidates are William Penn Abrams and U. N. Reamer, who were seeking possible lumber mill sites on the Merced in 1849. While bear hunting, they became lost and made their way north to what may be Old

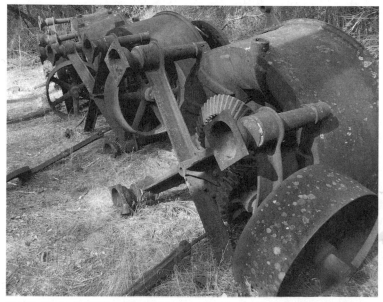

Historic equipment left at Hite's Cove

SAVAGE'S TRADING POST

The site of one of James Savage's trading posts is easy to visit. It is located on CA 140, 26 miles from Mariposa. The South Fork merges in from the east, and the site is now a motel. Nothing of the original trading post exists, but it is fun to imagine the early days. Adjacent to Savage's is a trail to Hite's Cove. In the 1860s John Hite's Native American wife led him to a spot where he mined out about $3 million in gold. Today the trail is managed by the U.S. Forest Service, and you can take the easy hike from CA 140 to see Hite's Cove.

Inspiration Point on the south rim of the valley. Abrams's journal, found in 1947, records his description of many key valley features, including Half Dome.

Gold Fever

The growth of the white population in California grew through the 1840s without much exploration of the Sierra. Arrivals came by ship from the East Coast, while others came over land via the lower, safer southern route. To provide lumber for the growing population, John Sutter ventured into the forested foothills of the Sierra east of Sacramento to set up a sawmill. He planned to get rich by selling the raw material, lumber, to feed the coming building boom. In January of 1848, while working at Sutter's Coloma sawmill (50 miles east of Sacramento), James Marshall came upon shiny flakes of gold. He showed them to Sutter, who decided to keep it quiet until work on a flour mill was finished. However, word leaked out, and a certain shopkeeper named Samuel Brannan in San Francisco heard the news and saw the opportunity to sell shovels, pans, and jeans. He ran though the streets of the city shouting "Gold! Gold! Gold from the American River!"

History tells the rest. Men across the country dropped every-thing and flocked to the foothills in droves. Ships sailed around the horn with anxious easterners ready to stake claims. To speed transit, a railroad was built across Panama. The gold rush was on. Rivers and streams were rerouted to reveal their rich beds; giant sluice boxes sprung up. Towns with names such as Angels Camp, Nevada City, Hornitos, Mariposa, and Garrote (Groveland) became household words. Today's CA 49 is littered with places that were once thriving gold towns. Sacramento boomed as supply stores, assay offices, banks, and brothels sprung up to support the miners. Newly rich miners found their way to San Francisco to relax and were quickly separated from their money. While many made small fortunes pulling out placer gold (the kind lying in streams), most of the real money was made by dry-goods sellers such as Brannan.

The 1846–1848 Mexican-American War gave California to the United States. Reflective of the boom, California was made a state on September 9, 1850. Many of the men who did not get lucky or hire on with bigger mining companies decided they liked California's terrain, weather, and freedom and settled in the foothills. Many began farming or working in support industries. It's relevant to note that during this time, because gold is usually not found in high mountains, there was no reason for further exploration to the east. The High Sierra remained unexplored and Yosemite was unknown.

Relations between the local tribes and the nonnatives became tense. The Native Americans were upset at the whites moving in. Some of the chiefs proposed that if the miners would give them some of the gold found on their lands, they could remain. The whites refused. The majority of the whites treated the natives as though they had no rights to be respected. Often, Native Americans who were working good mining claims were driven away by white miners, who then took possession of their claims and worked them. The Native Americans' main sources of food supply were being eliminated by the whites as well. Their diet of acorns was impacted as oak trees were cut down and burned by miners. Land was cleared for crops, and deer and other game were being killed off or driven off by farmers. Tensions escalated—the Native Americans began stealing horses and then began a series of attacks on trading posts. The raid of James Savage's trading post at the confluence of the Merced and the South Fork of the Merced spurred the locals to petition John McDougal, the governor of the new state, for help. In a letter to the governor dated January 13, 1851, Major James Burney, sheriff of Mariposa County, described the situation:

> *They have invariably murdered and robbed all the small parties they fell in with between here and the San Joaquin. News came here last night that seventy-two men were killed on Rattlesnake Creek; several men have been killed in Bear Valley. The Fine Gold Gulch has been deserted, and the men came in here yesterday. Nearly all the mules and horses in this part of the State have been stolen, both from the mines and the ranches. And I now in the name of the people of this part of the State, and for the good of our country, appeal to Your Excellency for assistance.*

This resulted in the formation of the volunteer Mariposa Battalion. James Savage, mentioned earlier, became captain and led the volunteer group. While Federal Indian Commissioners were negotiating with tribes to relocate to reservations along the Fresno River, the soldiers pursued Native Americans who refused to cooperate. During the winter of 1850–1851, they chased a band believed to live farther north. The resultant events were dubbed the Mariposa Indian War. It was on March 27, 1851, that they entered what we now call the Yosemite Valley.

The definitive source for the events of the Mariposa Indian War can be found in the Lafayette Houghton Bunnell, MD book *Discovery of the Yosemite, and the Indian War of 1851, which led to that event.* Bunnell was the medical man for the battalion. He wrote his book 30 years after the events because he felt too many magazines and newspapers were "getting it wrong."

The whites were impressed with what they saw. The soldiers learned much from Chief Tenaya, the leader of the Ahwahneechee, who were made up of renegades from various tribes. The soldiers wanted to honor the Native Americans by naming the place after them. Unfortunately, they mistakenly thought the locals were called the "Yo-Semite." It seems that through Native American interpreters, the soldiers confused the Sierra Miwok name *uz-mati,* or "grizzly bear," with a collective noun *yose-met-i,* meaning "the killers" or "a band of killers." The soldiers thought this meant "they are killers of grizzlies"—the bear that lived there. Chief Tenaya said that the name had been given to his band because they occupied the mountains and valleys, which were the favorite habitat of grizzly bears, and his people were expert in killing them. In actuality, the people who lived in the Yosemite Valley called it Ahwahnee. They referred to themselves as the Ahwahneechee. This error is easily understandable since the whites were unfamiliar with the language. Yo-Semite (now Yosemite) was used by early California geologist Josiah Whitney. The soldiers also tried to use Native American names for the rock formations, waterfalls, and sites, but the multisyllabic words were too much for later visitors to master. So today we have Vernal Fall not Yan-o-pah; Bridalveil Fall not Pohono; Yosemite Falls not Cholock; Mirror Lake not

Ahwiyah; El Capitan not Tote-ack-ah-noo-la; and Half Dome not Tissiack. The spelling of these Native American words is a guess, as they had no written language. After Tenaya's death in 1853, the remaining Yosemite Native Americans dispersed and Yosemite Valley became a white man's settlement.

The Crush Begins

Soon after its discovery, entrepreneurs entered the scene and began to promote Yosemite as a tourist destination. In 1855 James Hutchings led the first organized commercial tours in the valley. He kindled interest through his writings in his illustrated work *Hutchings' California Magazine*. Soon artists such as Thomas Hill, Thomas Ayres, and photographers such as Carleton Watkins came to record the wonderful sights for anxious eastern audiences. In the early years, great men, such as Eadweard Muybridge, J. J. Reilly, C. L. Pond, Charles Bierstadt,

Being an educated man, Lafayette Bunnell led the naming of many places in the valley. In his book he states:

As I did not take a fancy to any of the names proposed, I remarked that "an American name would be the most appropriate;" that "I could not see any necessity for going to a foreign country for a name for American scenery— the grandest that had ever yet been looked upon. That it would be better to give it an Indian name than to import a strange and inexpressive one; that the name of the tribe who had occupied it, would be more appropriate than any I had heard suggested." I then proposed "that we give the valley the name of Yo-sem-i-ty, as it was suggestive, euphonious, and certainly American; that by so doing, the name of the tribe of Indians which we met leaving their homes in this valley, perhaps never to return, would be perpetuated."

Charles L. Weed, and George Fiske, brought images of the park to eager audiences. Sadly, many photos and negatives are lost to time due to the many fires that happened at Yosemite.

Yosemite was charted by the U.S. Geologic Survey of California in 1863. Early visitors originally called Half Dome "South Dome" because they felt it balanced North Dome across the valley. Over the years, it has been called Cleft Rock, the Rock of Ages, and a few others that did not stick. However, Half Dome was soon the common name.

To help protect the pristine environs from commercial interests, in June 1864 President Abraham Lincoln signed the Yosemite Grant, which deeded Yosemite Valley and the Mariposa Grove of Big Trees (at the southern end) to the state of California. The bill mandated that this land be used for resort and recreation "for all time." The grant was overseen by the Yosemite Board of Commissioners, which was led by landscape architect Frederick Law Olmsted. Galen Clark was the first caretaker of the park. Note that only those two tracts of land were set aside for California to manage; the U.S. government retained the rest. John Muir arrived in 1868, and his writings influenced the country so much that, in 1890, Yosemite obtained federal protection as a national park. At that time the park was comprised only of the land *not* in the Yosemite Grant. Yosemite Valley and the Mariposa Grove of Big Trees were left under California jurisdiction. In 1905 the legislature of California re-granted Yosemite Valley and the Mariposa Grove back to the U.S. government. Congress accepted the state grant in 1906 and added these lands to Yosemite National Park. The completion of the transcontinental railroad in 1869 at Promontory, Utah, provided a fast way for people to get to the west, and the park continued to grow in the 1900s. Today attendance approaches 4 million visitors annually.

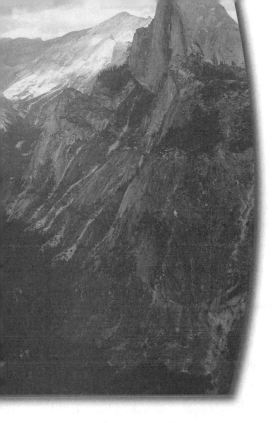

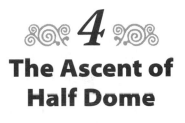

4

The Ascent of Half Dome

No one conquers Half Dome;
Tissiack lets you pass.

—Rick Deutsch

Since the whites entered the valley in 1851, they dreamed of getting to the top of Half Dome. There are no indications that any Native Americans ever made it to the top. In 1869 Josiah Whitney, the chief geologist for California, looked up and said, Half Dome is "perfectly inaccessible, being probably the only one of all the prominent points about the Yosemite which never has been, and never will be, trodden by human foot."

Many early settlers attempted to scale the 45-degree back side of Half Dome, including James Hutchings and Charles Weed in 1859. They brought Weed's photography gear but were unable to ascend the steep mountain. In the early 1870s John Muir's climbing buddy, expert climber George Bayley, also tried with the same result. This shows the difficulty of the task; Bayley was later the first to reach the top of Mount Starr King. Perhaps John Conway's sons got the closest. In September 1873

Conway, who also later crafted many trails at Yosemite, had his young sons attempt the feat. Led by 9-year-old Major Conway, the lizardlike boys, as described by John Muir, scrambled barefoot up the rock and inserted steel rods into cracks to which they attached a rope. Major reached an elevation of about 300 feet above the saddle, but father John mercifully called him back when he reached a steep point where he could find no projection to attach the rope.

It was just five years after Whitney's proclamation that George Anderson, a Scottish immigrant and former sailor, set out to top the mountain. Third-party accounts and writings years after the event have blurred the facts, but we believe Anderson quietly set up his work area in a small cabin he built nearby (the location has not been discovered but is believed to have been near a stream on the east side of the current Half Dome trail). Another cabin, where Anderson later lived at Foresta, is now on display at the Pioneer Yosemite History Center in Wawona.

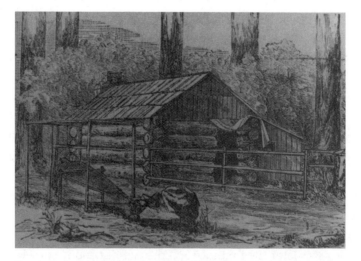

George Anderson's cabin at the foot of Half Dome;
credit: The Pacific Rural Press, 1881.

Working alone, he brought his forging station up and crafted dozens of 7-inch iron eyebolts on-site.

Anderson ascended Sub Dome and began his quest using remnants of the Conway rope. He pulled himself up as far as he could safely manage. Using a method called single jacking, he held a chisel and hit it with a hammer to drill shallow holes (about 0.5 inch wide and 6 inches deep) into the granite.

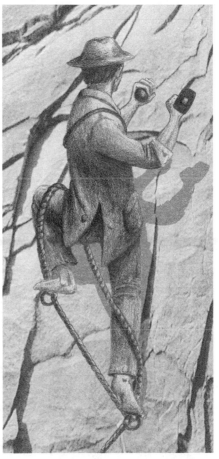

He slid small wooden pegs into the holes and then hammered in the eyelet spikes. They were placed about 5 feet apart. Next, he attached a rope to the eyelet and himself in case of a fall. He had to balance himself and stand on one spike to drill the hole for the next spike above. Each spike only stuck out about 2 inches. Up and up he went, building a crude ladder with about 40 of these eyebolts. Occasionally, some irregularity in the curve of the rock or slight foothold would enable him to free-climb 20 or so feet independently of the rope. He progressed more than 450 feet up the sloping granite, belayed only by the rope he tied to the spikes.

Once his spikes and pilot rope were in place, he returned to the valley to rig up a more sturdy rope. He modified a

900-foot-long rope by knotting five strands together with a sixth strand and a 3-inch sailor's knot a foot apart to allow a hand-over-hand traverse. This was a convenient space for future climbers to grasp as they made the ascent. Anderson used his mule to haul the new rope up to his cabin, and he carried it to the top using the spike ladder. He tied one end to the uppermost spike and slowly uncoiled and attached the rope to the eyelets with lashings. Although it was a crude device, it worked. At 3 p.m. on October 12, 1875, he erected a crude flagstaff and stood on top of Half Dome, "waving the starry flag of his adopted homeland," according to the *Mariposa Gazette*.

During all this, his shoes proved to be too slick, so he tried wearing just his socks, and then he wore bags coated with pine pitch tied below his knees; however, the pine pitch was too sticky to allow progress. He then tried wearing moccasins with pine pitch only on the soles. This technique appeared to work best and enabled him to adhere firmly to the smooth granite. But again, while the pitch prevented him from slipping, it also required great effort to move his feet and almost proved fatal several times. He settled on barefoot. Think of the pain of standing on 2 inches of the spike while balancing and hitting a sledgehammer to drill another hole. Pure determination. The way to the 13-acre summit was now in place. We don't know exactly how long all this took Anderson; estimates of a month seem reasonable. Each day he would work long and hard, and then return to his cabin area to forge new spikes and sharpen his chisel.

In the valley, Anderson's absence had been noticed and there was concern. A search party was sent up to look for him. On the trail near Nevada Fall, Anderson encountered the men and informed them he had reached the summit. The news quickly spread.

In the days following, he escorted several English tourists up the mountain. Soon after, he took up Galen Clark and Sally Dutcher, who became the first woman to climb to the top.

John Muir is believed to have been the ninth person on Half Dome. Muir later wrote of his November 10, 1875, experience in his books *The Mountains of California* and *The Yosemite,* as well as the November 18, 1875, edition of San Francisco's *Daily Evening Bulletin,* excerpted below:

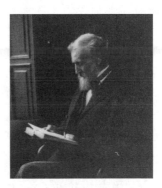

On my return to the valley the other day I immediately hastened to the Dome, not only for the pure pleasure climbing in view, but to see what else I might enjoy and learn. Our first winter storm had bloomed and all the mountains were mantled in fresh snow. I was therefore a little apprehensive of danger from slipperyness of the rock, Anderson himself refusing to believe that any one could climb his rope in the condition it was then in. . . . I therefore pushed up alone and gained the top without the slightest difficulty. My first view was perfectly glorious. A massive cloud of a pure pearl lustre was arched across the valley, from wall to wall, the one end resting upon El Capitan, the other on Cathedral Rocks, the brown meadows shadowed beneath, with short reaches of the river shimmering in changeful light. Then, as I stood on the tremendous verge overlooking Mirror Lake, a flock of smaller clouds, white as snow, came swiftly from the north, trailing over the dark forests, and arriving on the brink of the valley descended with godlike gestures through Indian Canyon and over the Arches and North Dome, moving rapidly, yet with perfect deliberation. . . .

I have always discouraged as much as possible every project for laddering the South Dome, believing it would be a fine thing to keep this garden untrodden. Now the pines will be carved with the initials of Smith and Jones, and the gardens strewn with tin cans and bottles, but the winter gales will blow most of this rubbish away, and avalanches may strip off the ladders; and then it is some satisfaction to feel assured that no lazy person will ever trample these gardens.

Anderson's feat planted the seeds of the big-wall climbing mecca that Yosemite has become. His climb marked the debut of bolt placements in the American climbing scene. It opened an inaccessible mountain to many Yosemite visitors and made Half Dome a destination for hiking and climbing enthusiasts from all over the world.

Yet Anderson did not rest on his laurels. He presented the idea of building a wooden staircase to the Yosemite Board of Commissioners. They set aside $2,000 for the project, but nothing came of it. Anderson even talked of building a steam-powered tram to take his guests to the top.

In the months that followed, others tried Anderson's route. However, the elements took their toll on the rope until it became unusable in a few years.

In the spring of 1884 Anderson died of pneumonia and was buried under a granite rock in the park cemetery. With Anderson gone, the hope was that "some venturesome member of the English Alpine Club should come along and have the goodness to replace it," as Alden Sampson wrote in a letter to author James M. Hutchings. Enter two true cowboys of the era, Sampson and A. Phimister Proctor. They arrived at Yosemite in search of fishing and relaxation and a try at going up Half

Dome. When they heard that a Brit was being sought to replace the rope, Sampson said: "This aspect of the matter, I must own, galled our pride; and the more we thought it over the less we liked this solution of the difficulty. Should we, forsooth, wait for foreign sinew to scale for us a peak of the American Sierras? Not if it lay in our power to prevent so humiliating a favor!"

After a short rest below Nevada Fall, at La Casa Nevada hotel, they rode their horses up the trail and arrived at Sub Dome to survey the situation. They saw that most of the original Anderson spikes had come out, making it difficult to ascend the smooth, steep sides. Being skilled cowboys, they used a rope to lasso higher spikes and rock holds. Proctor took the lead. The technique was to lasso a spike and then pull himself up. Amazingly, he did this barefoot because his cob nail boots were cutting in. Showing immense strength, he then did a jackknife to put his toe on the spike and worked his hand out. He would

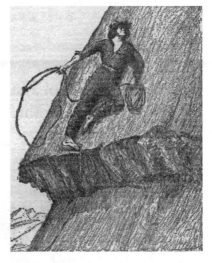

A. Phimister Proctor; courtesy A. Phimister Proctor Museum

A. Phimister Proctor went on to become a world-class bronze sculptor. His focus was on life-size animal- and western-themed monumental designs. His Teddy Roosevelt and buckaroo renderings are among my favorites. The Buffalo Bill Historical Center in Cody, Wyoming, houses many of Proctor's artworks, and the Proctor Museum in Seattle continues to preserve his legacy.

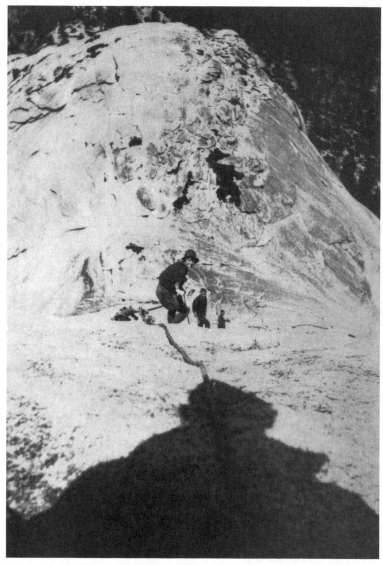

Vintage photo of the single rope system;
courtesy of the Yosemite Research Library, NPS

then lean precariously into the rock. All went well until they approached a bare stretch of a hundred feet, where every pin had been carried away. Gently clutching shrubs 8 inches high, the two gingerly hugged the rock. After many tries, Proctor finally snagged a rock edge and pulled himself up. They then were able to bring up their rope and secure it. Half Dome was open once more! However, the Proctor-Sampson rope also suffered from the harsh winters and soon became unusable. A replacement rope was installed by Thomas Magee Jr. and Stewart Rawlings in 1895, but it also frayed. Ropes put up in 1901 and later were successful to varying degrees.

Looking for attractions to draw tourists to his Camp Curry, David Curry pressed for an easier route to the top. In 1910 the Sierra Club placed a single rope down Half Dome's slope and removed the older ropes.

Ascents continued off and on, depending on the condition of the rope. On August 7, 1915, Arthur "A. C." Pillsbury led a group of 17 young Stanford students (including 6 women) up the back side of Half Dome. They used the rope remnants from previous explorers, their own rope, and a few of the George Anderson spikes that were still present from his first ascent in 1875. The group improved the route by placing a new half-inch Manila rope from top to bottom. Pillsbury snapped photos and motion pictures on top. He reportedly was suspended by rope to take some of the photos. Pillsbury was a Stanford graduate who had a studio in Yosemite. In his career, he invented key photographic tools, including the circuit panorama, the time-lapse, the microscopic motion picture, the X-ray motion picture, and the underwater motion picture cameras.

Construction of the Cable Route

M. Hall McAllister, a San Franciscan friend of John Muir and a member of the Sierra Club, offered to fund the erection of two steel cables to the summit of Half Dome. Upon approval of the project by the National Park Service, the contractor selected to design the cable route was Gutleben Brothers Construction Company, also of San Francisco. Christian and Dan Gutleben ran a project engineering company for industrial, government, corporate, and private construction projects. They did a lot of work for Yosemite from 1916 to 1926 and were involved in the Glacier Point Hotel, Yosemite Creek Bridge, Sentinel Bridge, the museum, the administration building, and other park buildings. Dated February 1919, and done by Christian Gutleben himself, their engineering drawing of the project, called the "Half Dome Stairway," is revealing.

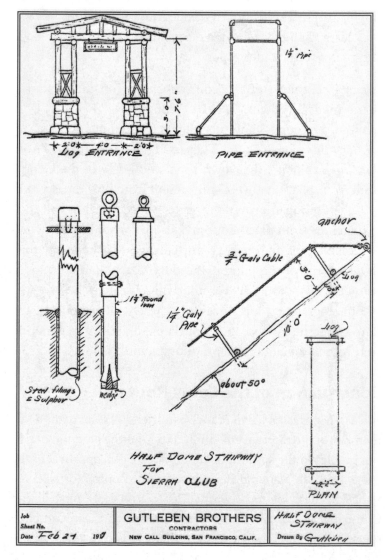

Plans for the cable route

At the left center of the plan you can see their ideas for the stations to hold up the cables. The intent was to fix the pipes permanently, but a major avalanche in 1919–1920 ripped out many of the pipes. In subsequent years, the removable pipes were installed and remain today. The right side of the drawing clearly shows the actual cable installation, with 0.75-inch cables held up by 3-foot galvanized pipes with a 1.25-inch diameter. The pipes are 10 feet apart with logs instead of today's 2-by-4-foot wooden footrests. Note that the angle is listed at an imprecise "about 50 degrees."

The actual drilling work for the support pipes on Half Dome was done by the McGilvrey Brothers. The steel cables were carried up all the way to the Sub Dome by mules. As part of

The cables

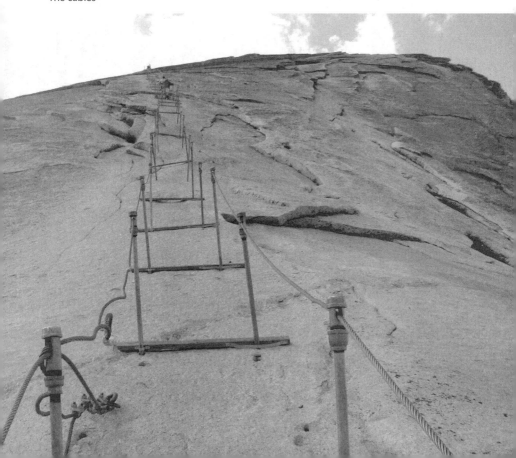

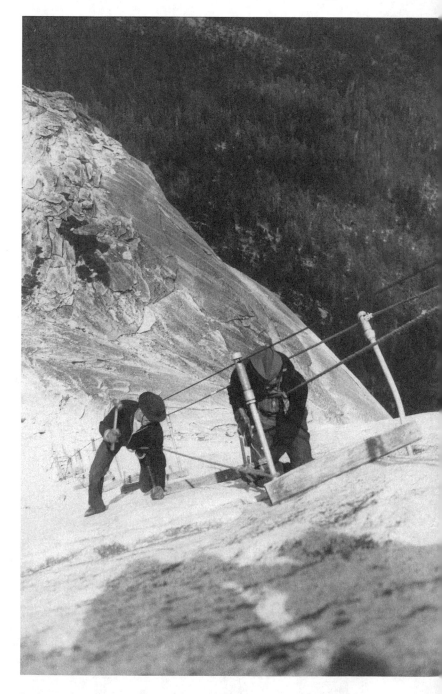

Replacing the cables in 1934; courtesy of the Yosemite Research Library, NPS the project, steps were added to the Sub Dome (these were improved in 1972, 1982, and 2005). The project was completed in time for the summer 1919 season. Total cost was $4,357.57, with McAllister giving more than $3,700 for labor and material. The park provided $300 in tools and related equipment. Transportation costs ran about $270. At completion, the system was turned over to the NPS for the use of all. What we use today are not the original cables, so there is no historic value to them. The Civilian Conservation Corps replaced them in 1934, and the NPS did so again in 1984.

In honor of George Anderson's singular accomplishment, it was felt that an entrance gateway at Sub Dome should be built. The arch was completed, and a sign directing visitors to a water source and a plaque honoring Anderson were installed. The plaque read:

ERECTED 1919 UNDER THE AUSPICES
OF THE SIERRA CLUB
TO REMEMBER
CAPTAIN GEORGE ANDERSON
WHO FIRST ASCENDED THIS DOME IN 1875

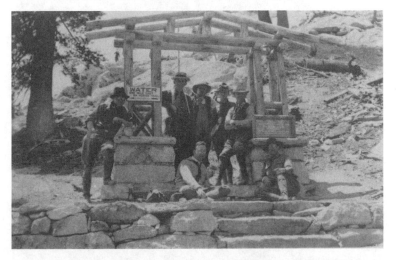

The Anderson Memorial Arch at the base of Sub Dome; courtesy of the Yosemite Research Library, NPS

You can still see the stone block remnants of the base of the arch where the rangers check for permits. Being made of wood, the arch didn't last long in the rough winters of the Sierra.

The Slippery Slope

The cables allow a vertical ascent of 425 feet. This is easily measured by using a GPS device. To confirm the slope, I took up a hardware store inclinometer to measure the degrees of incline of the rocks from horizontal along the cable route. While not super accurate, it was at least a first cut. A week prior, I used an iPhone clinometer app to do the measurements. This proved very difficult, as I had no way to secure the device to me and risked dropping it. The reflective face of the iPhone had a lot of glare and was very hard to read. Plus, it took many seconds for the digital display to stabilize. All this while I was hanging onto the cable hunched over. I was getting very high readings—in the mid-50 degrees. I decided this was not efficient or safe and that I should return later with the hardware store unit.

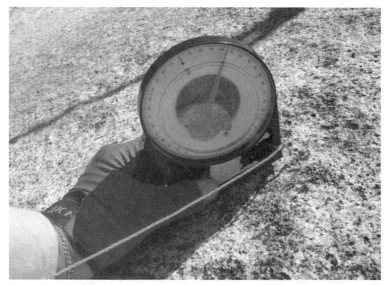

Measuring the slope

To try to get impartial readings, I placed the inclinometer between pole sets and took 40 readings. I began at the bottom where the incline is mellow. The slope gradually increased from 33, 35, 37, to 40 degrees at the first anchor point. Continuing up I recorded a steady slope of 44 degrees with a peak of 46 degrees at the second anchor point. From there, it held at about 44, then gradually came down into the mid-30s. At the final upper anchor point it read 34 degrees.

This is an admittedly crude measure because the rock is rough and I may have placed the device such that irregularities in the rock over- or under-recorded the slope. But it was a first attempt. The ultimate solution is an integral calculus problem, and an accurate answer would entail recording hundreds of points with a device that had an extremely small

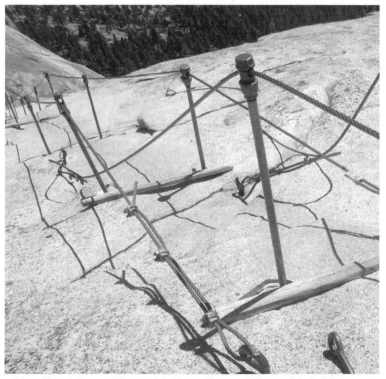

Anchor point; cable transition

base. Using my method, I found that the slope grew steeper from 31 degrees to a maximum of 46 degrees about halfway to the top. It certainly feels greater than 46 degrees, but I did not record any steeper with the 40 data points. I did this on my descent and had the inclinometer strung to my belt and bent down to the rock to view the reading after several seconds to stabilize the needle.

If you approximate the slope at 45 degrees, then the total run of the cables can be found using simple trigonometry assuming a right triangle. Applying the Pythagorean theorem, the total length traversed is a bit over 600 feet. I do know of one attempt at a tape measurement using a 100-foot tape measure. In that effort, they came up with a measurement of 797 feet. I spoke with the team who did it, and they confessed the tape had a lot of kinks in it and was very unwieldy, so they may have been off. Plus, the start and end points need to be verified.

Each of the two cables is actually assembled in thirds, with each run anchored to the granite rock. The cables are held upright by 68 pairs of 3-foot pipes placed into 5-inch holes drilled into the rock. To allow a hiker to stand vertical, 2-by-4-foot boards are loosely fastened to the pipes.

The pipes and boards are put in place by the NPS trail crew every late May (weather permitting) and are removed in early October (usually after Columbus Day). It takes about 20 skilled people to carefully handle the pipes and boards. They are secreted away in the off-season.

The cables themselves remain on the mountain year-round. Although not prohibited, it is not advised to ascend Half Dome during the off-season unless you are a skilled big-wall climber. It is very dangerous to use only the cable to rappel up and down. When the rock has any moisture on it, it is very slippery.

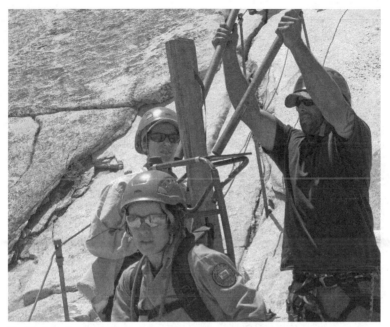

Modified backpacks hold the hardware; courtesy of NPS/Joy Marschall

People have fallen when using the cable without the pipes and poles in place. (See Appendix 3, Accidents, for details.)

Half Dome Today

The top surface consists of a few large hunks of granite at the north peak and a smooth, sloping area toward Curry Village. Depending how you measure, the top is about 13 acres or 17 football fields.

The north wall dominates that edge. Muir wrote of the wild-flowers and seven pine trees on the top. Early visitors cut down most for firewood, so today only one gnarled large shrub is left. Surprisingly, there are many wildflowers and small plants to see. Marmots and squirrels appear to be the only inhabitants. These furry mammals are cute, but resist the temptation to feed them.

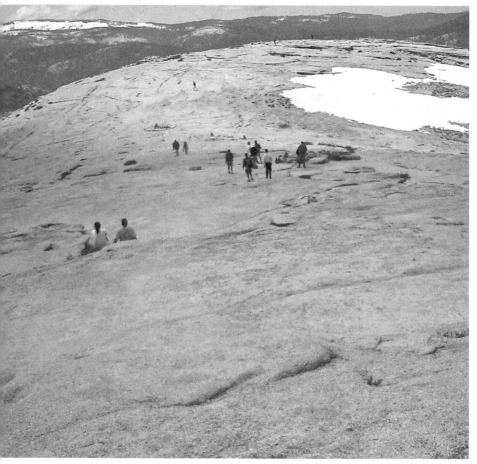

Half Dome is surprisingly large up top with snow in June

Currently more than 40,000 people attempt the Half Dome hike each year. Most are successful. With the thousands of visitors who reach the summit each year, I was surprised to find that there is no formal control over who can go up the cables. Age, size, and strength don't matter. No one monitors the cables, so if you are willing, you can attempt the ascent. This reflects the personal freedom we enjoy in America. I'm often asked about the oldest or youngest person who has gone up the cables. No records are kept. Most kids are about 10 years old at the youngest (although younger have gone up), and I know of people over 80 who have made the ascent. (Again, no formal records are kept, so don't risk safety by going for a record.) Please make a rational decision about taking children. This is a hard hike and children especially need to be properly outfitted and prepared. They should be allowed to rest often and go at their pace—not yours. Water is essential for them. Turn back if it becomes too hard; don't push them.

Half Dome is also known for its oft-photographed 2,000-foot sheer face. Rock climbers can scale it in 3–4 days. It is one of the world's most vertical rock walls. It was first climbed in 1957 by Royal Robbins, Mike Sherrick, and Jerry Gallwas (all then in their early 20s), taking them five days. The record for an ascent was set in June 2008 by Alex Honnold, who free-climbed (no ropes or supports and alone) in 2 hours 50 minutes. Today, this wall and nearby El Capitan are popular climbs; however, our undertaking is a hike and not a climb. We will venture up the safer back side of Half Dome.

The requirement for permits began in 2010. This was an interim process to help alleviate the congestion on the cables and to provide a solution to potential bottlenecks on the cables

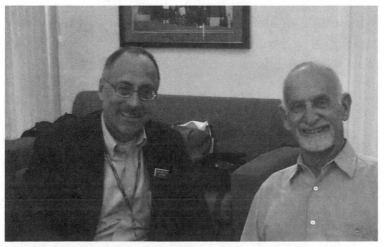

Mr. Half Dome (left) meets Royal Robbins

Half Dome was declared part of Yosemite's designated wilderness by the U.S. Congress in 1984. In the valley, the boundary is the 4,200-foot mark, but it also stretches up the Merced corridor to the top of Nevada Fall. This allows visitors to enjoy a spirit of adventure, discovery, and some risk. Accordingly, visitors must assess the risk of their actions and deal with it appropriately. No ranger will make judgment as to your ability to ascend Half Dome, nor will he or she give any approval or prohibit you from going up. A ranger may advise you as to the conditions but will not stop you. It is totally *your* decision to proceed or not. Do not go up if there is any chance of inclement weather. People have died when lightning, hail, rain, or damp conditions exist. The rock will be there for a future trip. You are not permitted to camp on top. This was ended in 1992 due to human impact and because it is the habitat of the endangered Mount Lyell salamander. It lives deep in the cracks and is seldom seen. When campers would build wind shelters using the rocks, they disturbed the animals. You cannot camp above 7,900 feet in the Half Dome region.

when weather suddenly changes for the worse. In addition, permits allow for a much better experience for hikers. This topic will be discussed in detail in Chapter 7, Preparation.

Overview of the Half Dome Hike

Why would you want to hike up to Half Dome? The quick answer is: "Because it's there!" Seriously, after one has done the other challenging valley hikes, such as Yosemite Falls, Clouds Rest, or Glacier Point, there comes a time to enter into the fraternity of those who "made it to the top," as the gift store T-shirt says. Half Dome is a grand accomplishment. Doing anything for 10–12 hours is cause for celebration. The hike can awaken your adventuresome spirit with a new feeling of self confidence. For many people, this is their Mount Everest and is one of the most ambitious things they will ever undertake. Maybe after conquering Half Dome you'll embark on even more challenging adventures. Perhaps California's Mount Whitney or Mount Shasta, the Milford Track in New Zealand, Kilimanjaro in Tanzania, or Machu Picchu in Peru are on your list.

The Half Dome hike is a first-class adventure. You'll get up close and personal with Vernal Fall and Nevada Fall, stroll through scenic Little Yosemite Valley, and view the crystal-clear Merced River. The long series of switchbacks on the way to the base of Half Dome are strenuous and will test your resolve to get to the top. Finally, there is the long pull up the cables, which is guaranteed to raise your heart rate. All of this will lead you to the climax: standing on the very top of Half Dome and gazing down nearly a mile onto the valley floor.

Some people do this hike in two days. They load backpacks, hike up one day, and arrive in Little Yosemite Valley to spend the night (permit required). Then the next morning they summit with a smaller daypack and return to the valley floor the same day. My preference is for a one-day hike. Carrying a 30- to 40-pound pack up the steep trails is quite a lot of work. Although you'll enjoy the fun of the camping experience, you'll also need to deal with bears. You'll have to carry all your food, clothing, and gear about 2,000 feet up from the valley. A one-day trip is very doable. You'll need an early start; before 6 a.m. is recommended. For a one-day trip, you will need to carry only minimal equipment, as described later. Your hike will start out chilly but should soon warm up to be pleasant. With increasing altitude the air will actually get cooler (you will lose 3°F for every 1,000 feet you ascend). If you keep a good pace, you should be heading up the cables well before noon and will arrive back to your camp before sunset. (Bring a flashlight, just in case.)

When you're on the top, a few feet from the edge, you can look down on the Ahwahnee Hotel or over at Clouds Rest, Glacier Point, El Capitan, and toward the vast San Joaquin Valley in the distance. So this is why we do it. It's a tough view to equal. With education, preparation, and motivation, almost anyone can do it. Seize the day!

Leave No Trace

I highly encourage you to respect Yosemite (and other areas you frequent) so that future generations can enjoy them too. The "leave no trace" principles are merely common-sense outdoor ethics to help preserve our fragile ecosystem. Leave no trace is an awareness and an attitude, not a rigid set of rules. As more natural areas are turned into strip malls and parking lots, humans need places to go for respite and to contemplate the meaning of life. Keep these principles in mind:

1. Plan ahead and prepare.
2. Travel and camp on durable surfaces.
3. Dispose of waste properly.
4. Leave what you find.
5. Minimize campfire impacts.
6. Respect wildlife.
7. Be considerate of other visitors.

Hiking is a fun, rewarding, and healthy experience. You'll soon join a strong community of hikers. I find it interesting that folks say "hello" as they pass on a trail, yet put up a protective shield if they see the same person in a store. Be courteous when passing others on a trail and always let downhill hikers have the right-of-way on a narrow passage. They will have momentum, and yielding to them will give you a chance to rest!

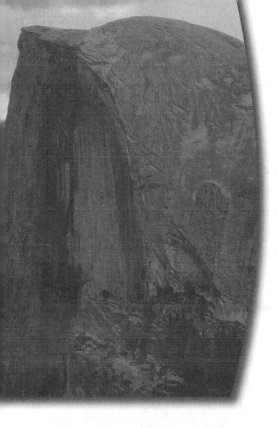

5
Precautions

The clearest way into the Universe
is through a forest wilderness.

—John Muir

This is basically a very safe hike; however, a few words of caution are appropriate. Make sure you understand the challenge ahead of you. Do not attempt the hike if you are not prepared.

Intensity

Of the 23 hikes listed in the official park guide, the Half Dome hike is the only one described as extremely strenuous. The raw facts speak volumes: about 16 miles round-trip, 10–12 hours in duration, and 4,737-foot altitude gain. Make sure that you're physically prepared for an adventure of this magnitude. If you've done your training, gotten in shape, and had a recent physical exam, you'll be fine. When's the last time you ever did anything for up to 12 continuous hours? Have you walked on a flat path for that long? Even sleeping 12 hours will make you sore! And your first attempt at hiking Half Dome may well take you longer than 12 hours.

Weather

Summer in Yosemite is pure heaven. The days are warm and dry, and the nights are cool. Mid- to late summer can bring very high temperatures to the valley, and your hike will become even more challenging. It's not unusual for August temperatures to approach 100°F. Fortunately, clear skies generally prevail, but an occasional shower is common in any mountain environment. For the Half Dome hike, you'll be limited to the summer season, consistent with the installation of the cable system. However, the biggest concern is lightning. Storms can arise at any time of year, but they are most common during the later summer months. In August, localized hot air often meets cooler upper-layer air, creating

LIGHTNING IS DEADLY

In July of 1985, five hikers ascended Half Dome late in the day and met with tragedy from two ferocious lightning strikes. Their story is documented in the book *Shattered Air: A True Account of Catastrophe and Courage on Yosemite's Half Dome,* by Bob Madgic. It recounts how the young men, full of enthusiasm and bravado, ignored nature's warnings and hiked up the famed cable trail right into the vortex of a fierce thunderstorm. They took shelter in the rock cave enclosure at the summit. Lightning struck the dome twice, killing one of the hikers and causing a second to tumble over the edge. Two survivors were gravely injured. Other hikers arrived at the scene and administered emergency medical treatment for more than five hours deep into the night. Finally, an air ambulance helicopter arrived in Yosemite Valley at 12:30 a.m. and, in a race with the descending moon, made three dangerous trips to the top of Half Dome to bring the surviving victims down from the summit.

cumulonimbus clouds and resulting in thunderstorms and lightning accompanied by heavy rains. You may be deceived, because days often start out clear and with blue skies. Slowly, clouds move in until the skies are overcast and you can hear distant thunder rumbling. Once the skies open up, storms usually last a few hours. Not only is it no fun slogging through mud, but it can be extremely dangerous. Slick and muddy footing can result in ankle twists and falls, but lightning can be deadly. If you hear any thunder, immediately turn around and return to the valley. Do not continue on your hike to Half Dome. The large granite rock is a giant lightning rod. Not only is the surface of the rock very slick when wet, making it nearly impossible to go up, but as one of the highest structures in the area, the rock attracts lightning strikes. People have been struck and have died as a result of lightning. Even if you have clear skies above, lightning can travel more than 10 miles from its source. A permanent sign at the base of Half

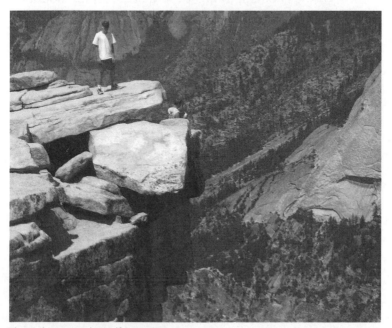

The rock cave on the Half Dome Visor

Dome cautions hikers not to ascend when thunder is in the area. On the very top of Half Dome is an outcrop of rocks, near the northwest peak. What looks like a cave is actually a jumble of large rock slabs near the Visor. This seems like it would be a safe haven in a storm. It's not.

If there's even a hint of thunder, lightning, or rain, get off the rock immediately and get to a lower elevation. Do not press your luck. Be nowhere near Half Dome if there is even a remote chance of adverse weather coming in. (It will be there to hike another day!) If you cannot immediately get down to a lower altitude, get away from tall trees, toss your hiking poles, and insulate yourself from the ground by squatting on your pack and presenting the smallest possible target for the lightning.

Altitude Sickness

The apex of Half Dome is at 8,842 feet, a height where altitude sickness is not commonly experienced. Acute mountain sickness (AMS) is usually only a concern well above this elevation. However, anyone who goes to higher altitudes can get AMS. Susceptibility is primarily related to individual physiology and genetics, as well as the rate of ascent. Age, gender, physical fitness, or previous altitude experience do not seem to be significant factors. Symptoms include headache, fatigue, weakness, dizziness, nausea, and stomach distress.

At the far end of the altitude sickness spectrum are high altitude cerebral edema (HACE) and high altitude pulmonary edema (HAPE). These are potentially life-threatening illnesses that usually do not occur below 12,000 feet. If you decide to follow up the Half Dome hike with an expedition to the top of Yosemite's 13,000-foot peaks or even to nearby Mount Whitney to the south (at 14,495 feet, it's the highest point in the lower 48), then you'll need to read up on HACE and HAPE. These are serious conditions, and discussing them is outside the scope of this book. Medical science has a lot to learn about altitude sickness, as it appears to be variable for each individual. If you're concerned, you can spend a day or two in the park doing some test hikes to get acclimated. If you do experience altitude sickness symptoms, the best cure is to descend. Drugs are rarely helpful. Getting a good night's sleep the day before the hike, drinking lots of water, and avoiding alcohol may reduce symptoms. In general, children are more susceptible to altitude sickness than adults. The rule of thumb is that if you feel unwell at altitude, it is probably altitude sickness unless there is another obvious explanation. The immediate action is to descend. Again, the good news is that Half Dome just isn't high enough to cause problems for most people.

Mosquitoes

Pesky mosquitoes congregate near water sources. At Yosemite, their presence depends a lot on the previous winter snowpack and when the melt occurs. Fortunately, you will see few of the critters on this hike thanks to the wind and the lack of standing water. You may get bitten while relaxing on the valley floor. The worst times will be in the morning and at dusk, when the air and water are calm. It's a good idea to apply a repellent and wear long pants and sleeves. An outdoor ranger talk or evening walk can be a challenge if you do not take precautions. Bugs are more of a problem in the backcountry and not so much on the Half Dome hike.

Ticks

In spring ticks become active. The species present in the park can transmit the bacteria that cause Lyme disease. Ticks prefer cool, moist environments, such as shrubs and grasses; for complete protection, avoid those places. Check yourself and others periodically. Wear light-colored clothing so that ticks stand out. It's a good idea to tuck your pants into your boots or socks.

Gaiters are handy to close the gap between your boots and pants. You may also want to spray repellent on your clothes. On the Half Dome trail, you'll be walking on gravel, dirt, or stones, so the odds of picking up a tiny hitchhiker are small.

Waterborne Critters

The days of dipping your canteen into the closest stream for a refreshing drink are pretty much gone in today's world. Water contaminated with bacteria, viruses, and protozoans can cause serious illness or even death. The U.S. Environmental Protection Agency has estimated that nearly 90% of the world's fresh water is contaminated. Giardiasis is a concern in Yosemite. It is caused through infection of the intestine by the single-celled parasite *Giardia lamblia.* Another harmful parasite called *Cryptosporidium* may also be in the water.

If ingested, these parasites live and reproduce in human or animal intestines. Once in the intestines, they attach to the inside of the intestinal wall, where they can disrupt the normal function of the intestines and compete for nutrients. They can survive for a long time in soil or water until they are ingested by another host. Giardia is spread by contact with the fecal matter of deer, rodents, bears, birds, and people. The risk is that you may end up with a range of discomforts, including severe diarrhea. Don't assume that because you find a natural stream you are safe. The same goes for the sparkling waters of the Merced. Some people think that if you dip into a moving water source, it's ok to drink. Wrong. Don't do it! The giardia protozoans can cause one of the more common types of dysentery, and you may not feel the effect until about 10 days after your trip. You may not even associate your illness with your hike. I had a friend who was sick for a long time. The doctors traced the possible cause to a day that he spent at Yosemite when he cooled himself off under a waterfall and swallowed some of the spray. The symptoms to watch out for include stomach pain, diarrhea, nausea, malaise, gas, and weight loss. If you suffer from these, get treatment. However, the parasite may not totally go away, and symptoms could erupt years later. Prevention methods (discussed in Chapter 7, Preparation, Water), such as filtration, UV light, boiling, and chemical tablets, are recommended. While the odds of getting sick are low, it's better to be on the cautious side.

It's also a good idea to clean your hands regularly, especially after using the toilet facilities and before eating. In order to avoid spreading germs, don't touch your face. Since the only potable water on the trail is at the Vernal Fall footbridge, hand cleaning is best accomplished with antibacterial wipes or gels. These are available in travel sizes and will greatly reduce the chance of illness.

The Falls

On this hike, you'll come close to two very high waterfalls. Although Yosemite Falls, at 2,425 feet, is the tallest in North America, two impressive falls on the trail will also amaze you. First, you'll reach Vernal Fall (317 feet), then later Nevada Fall (594 feet). Both are full and flowing in the spring as the winter snow melts. They are on the Merced River and offer great photo opportunities. If you arrive later in the summer, their flows will be quite reduced.

Sadly, occasionally someone goes over the falls accidentally. The area near the Vernal Fall footbridge is notorious for people slipping off the rocks. During the spring, Class V rapids flow. If a person falls, they are often trapped in the rock jumble and are not able to be found until the flow decreases. Rescue is nearly impossible because of the tremendous volume of water in high season. At the base of the falls, large boulders form caves that can trap a body. It is common for bodies to be pulled out more than a hundred yards downstream.

In July 2011, a tragedy occurred when three people climbed over the protective railing at Vernal Fall, slipped, and were washed over. The snowpack that year was about 200% of normal, and the falls flowed well into late summer. The falls

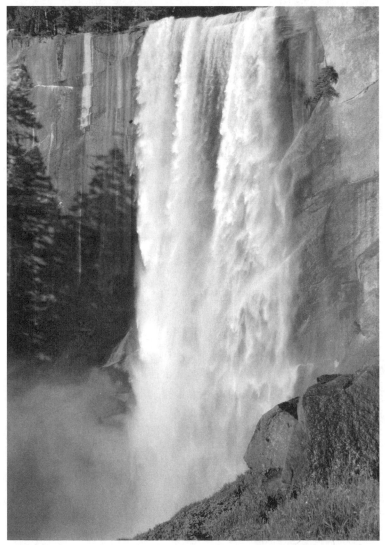

Vernal Fall

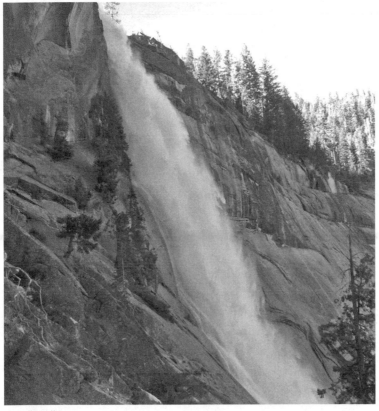

Nevada Fall

at Yosemite are all fed by melting snow and usually go dry by mid-July.

By late summer, the flow changes from a roaring cascade to a mere trickle. In fall and winter, it's interesting to view the bottom of one of the bigger falls. The jumbled collection of huge boulders confirms why immediate body recovery is very difficult. On the Half Dome hike, the waters above Vernal and Nevada falls are inviting. Venturing out from the shore is very risky because the current can knock you over while you stand on the smooth rocks. Once a person is in the cold, fast-moving waters, it is very difficult to get out. Be respectful of the Merced!

IS IT VERNAL FALL OR VERNAL FALLS?

While most of us are used to calling any waterfall "falls," there is a distinction. If the water generally goes over the edge straight down to the bottom without hitting rocks, it's called a singular fall. If there are intermediary stages (or cascades), it's called the plural falls, as in Yosemite Falls. To confuse things, if you were talking about Vernal Fall and Nevada Fall together, they would be "the falls."

Falling

Although most of this hike is mellow, there are stages where you'll encounter rough granite steps and challenging footing. You'll be on gravel and pointed rocks that may cause you to slip or trip. Always watch where you are stepping and be in control. Take your time. You'll need to ascend three very difficult stretches: the lower Mist Trail (about 700 steps), the upper Mist Trail (about 1,200 steps), and the approach just before the cables, called Sub Dome (about 500 steps).

Take your time and don't rush. If you lose your concentration on the trail, you risk taking a nasty fall. Sprained ankles and broken bones are among the most common injuries, but high-top boots will protect against ankle sprains, and hiking poles provide stability. The biggest technical challenge is climbing up (and down) the cables on the back side of Half Dome. This will definitely give you a rush. Be advised that although very rare, people have fallen to their deaths by slipping from the cables. A 2,000-foot drop looms not far from the cables. A wet surface, smooth-soled shoes, and a lost grip have been the primary causes of falls. If a person faints or suffers a heart attack, the stanchions and other hikers may stop his or her descent. If you feel at all queasy or light-headed, go back down. Ask others for help.

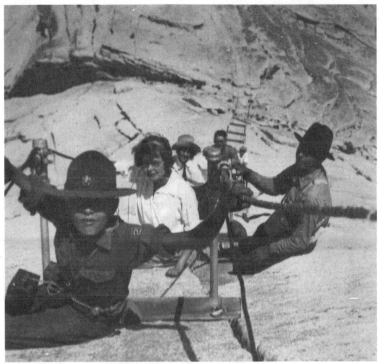

Boy Scout leads climb in 1924; courtesy Yosemite Museum NPS

The pull up the cables is much easier when you arrive before 11 a.m., when you should have a clear path with few people crowding you. Normally, this means leaving no later than 6 a.m. from the trailhead. The permit system has ended the crowding of previous years, which saw up to 1,200 people going up on a busy summer weekend day. Make sure that the trail is open to hiking on the days you want to go.

Wildlife

All park animals are wild; for your safety do not feed or touch them. Yosemite is home to a variety of wildlife. These are not pets—they are wild animals and should be treated with respect. There are bears, mountain lions, coyotes, scorpions, rattlesnakes, deer, bobcats, gray foxes, mountain beavers, great gray owls, white-headed woodpeckers, spotted owls, golden-mantled ground squirrels, martens, Steller's jays, pikas, yellow-bellied marmots, white-tailed hares, and more than 150 species of birds. Bighorn sheep formerly populated the Sierra crest but have been reduced to only a few remnant populations. Yosemite has more than 300 species of vertebrate animals, and 85 of these are native mammals. You might encounter some of these animals on your hike. All are protected and may not be hunted or harassed.

The biggest concern for many visitors is the bears. It's estimated that up to 500 black bears live within the park's boundaries. The term *black* is misleading because the actual color of these bears varies from blond to cinnamon brown to black. At more than 350 pounds, they can be big. The grizzly bear (as seen on the California state flag) is now extinct from the state. In Yosemite, the last one was killed in 1895.

Most bears in Yosemite live far from the valley, residing in the vast backcountry. The populated valley floor provides an easy meal for wandering bears. June–August, the bears normally eat currants, raspberries, chokeberries, and manzanita berries. When these are scarce, the bears may wander through campgrounds, looking for leftovers. Their superb sense of smell and intellect can guide them right to the cooler in your car. Cubs are often trained to climb trees to get to food bags. Bears recognize that boxes in the shape of coolers mean food. Empty soda cans and food wrappers might encourage a bear to examine the inside of your car further. Scented items such as sprays, suntan lotion, and even toothpaste might attract them. You can imagine the damage they can cause.

The National Park Service has an aggressive program to reduce human-bear contact. Bear-resistant canisters are highly effective and required in Yosemite National Park. Valley campers and car owners must sign a form showing that they understand the rules. The best solution is the use of bear boxes in the campsites and a vigorous education program. Please heed the advice you receive and help save an unwitting bear from expulsion or worse.

It is rare that you'll even see a bear on the Half Dome trail. In all my trips I've only seen two during the hike, and they were far off. If you do see one, leave it alone. Keep at least 50 yards away. If it is aggressive and you have a cell phone, call the park's Save-a-Bear hotline at (209) 372-0322 for the authorities to come and deal with it. If you see a bear at your campsite, make loud noises to scare it away. Look big, yell, and toss rocks near it. Bears are inherently shy and would prefer to avoid a confrontation. Finally, never try to play with cubs; they are cute, but momma won't like it and may want to teach you a lesson. In reality, more people at Yosemite are hurt by encounters with deer than with bears. In fact, the only fatality caused by wildlife was a 5-year-old boy who was gored by a deer. He was feeding a buck potato chips when things turned bad. No one has ever been killed by a bear at the park.

Mountain lions also populate Yosemite. Sightings are rare, but be aware of their existence. Humans are not their natural food,

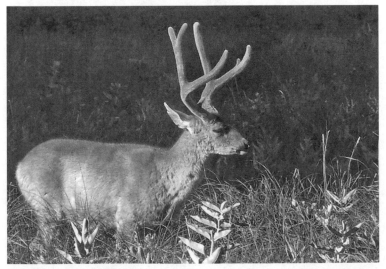

Mule deer

but the cats can be unpredictable. Don't hike alone and keep small children near you. If you encounter a lion, hold your ground or back away slowly. If it appears to be threatening you, wave your arms or hold your coat open. Your goal is to make yourself look as large and threatening as possible—but don't aggressively approach the lion. Maintain eye contact and do not crouch down. Do not run—this will ignite the lion's hunting instincts. If you sense an attack, throw sticks or rocks at the lion. Pick up or restrain small children to keep them from panicking and running. If a lion attacks, fight back!

Rattlesnakes are common in the park. The many rocky crevices make nice homes for them. If you wander off established trails or go bouldering, be aware of their presence. Do not reach into holes or between rocks. The snakes are not aggressive but can be territorial and could strike if you are probing where you should not. Fortunately, they make the distinctive rattle noise to warn you to back off. This is a good reason not to listen to music while hiking! In spring babies emerge. They are actually more of a problem than adults, as they will continue to bite while the adults bite once and then retreat. If you are bitten, remain calm, immobilize the bitten part of your body, and stay as quiet as possible to keep the poison from spreading through your body. Remove jewelry before you start to swell. Position yourself so that the bite is at or below the level of your heart. Cleanse the wound, but don't flush it with water, and cover it with a clean, dry dressing. Apply a splint to reduce movement of the affected area, but keep it loose enough so as not to restrict blood flow. Don't use a tourniquet or apply ice; don't cut the wound or attempt to remove the venom; don't drink caffeine or alcohol; and don't try to capture the snake. Do try to remember its color and shape so you can describe it, which will help in your treatment. Call 911 or seek a ranger to get help, especially if your skin changes color, begins to swell, or is painful.

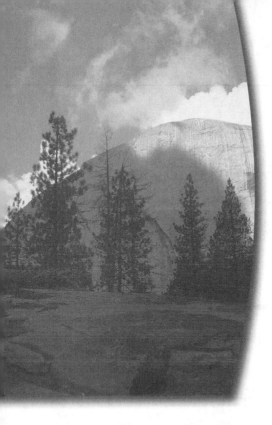

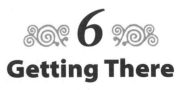

Getting There

Everybody needs beauty as well as bread, places to play in and pray in, where nature may heal and give strength to body and soul alike.

—John Muir

Yosemite is about 200 miles east of San Francisco, California. Half Dome is at 37° 44' 46" north latitude and 119° 31" 55" west longitude. From the Bay Area, the drive is an easy 3–4 hours, depending on your stops and observance of speed limits. Be advised that the California Highway Patrol (CHP) is one of the nation's finest and uses radar to monitor speed. The Los Angeles basin lies about 300 miles to the south, and visitors arrive in droves from that area as well. The drive from LA is about 6 hours. The only major population center to the north and east is Reno/Lake Tahoe. Most international visitors to Yosemite will probably arrive at the San Francisco, Sacramento, or Fresno airports. I suggest you consult an online map service for precise directions and travel times from your starting point. For your GPS, enter the zip code for the park as 95389. Distances in miles to the Yosemite Valley from major nearby cities are presented on the following page.

From	Miles	From	Miles
Bakersfield, CA	200	Oakdale, CA	110
Fresno, CA	90	Reno, NV	235
Groveland, CA	70	Sacramento, CA	190
Las Vegas, NV	425	San Diego, CA	430
Lee Vining, CA	95	San Francisco, CA	210
Los Angeles, CA	310	San Jose, CA	200
Mariposa, CA	60	Sonora, CA	90
Monterey, CA	220		

There are four access highways into the park. These are
California highways 120 (east and west), 41, and 140. All
are well-maintained roads but may be closed during winter
storms. CA 120 from Crane Flat through Tioga Pass is not
plowed until early summer.

Arriving via CA 41 Northbound

Southern California access to Yosemite is via CA 99 or I-5.
The turnoff at Kettleman City onto CA 41 features a sprawl-
ing (and odoriferous) cattle ranch (and super steak dinners!).
Continuing on, Fresno is a large metropolis for last-minute
shopping. Soon, CA 41 becomes a scenic mountainous road.
Oakhurst will be your last major gas and food stop, and you
can indulge at a nearby casino.

As you drive north, you will arrive at Fish Camp and the
Sugar Pine Railroad on your right. This is a fun diversion.
There you can learn about the importance of lumber in the
growth of the area. Sugar Pine has two historic Shay steam
locomotives, which were built in 1913 and 1928 and relocated
from Tuolumne. These locomotives are representative of the
machines that hauled lumber from 1874 to 1931.

Continuing north, you will enter the south entrance of the
park near Wawona and the Mariposa Grove. Galen Clark

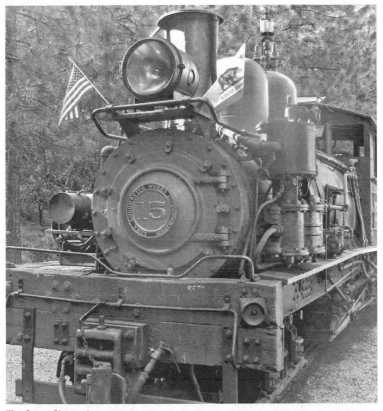

The Sugar Pine train

discovered these giants in 1857. Clark had moved from Philadelphia to Mariposa in 1854 to seek his fortune in gold. He suffered from tuberculosis and soon moved to the southern area of the park and built Clark's Station as a rest stop for visitors going to the valley. While hunting he came upon the tree cluster that we now call the Mariposa Grove of Big Trees (Giant Sequoias)—some of the world's tallest trees. Plan extra time to see the big trees. Walking access is easy from the parking lot.

After traveling 4 miles into the park, you need to stop at the famous Wawona Hotel. Built in 1876 by the Washburn brothers, it was an outgrowth of Clark's Station. The original hotel suffered a major fire in 1878 but was rebuilt to its present 104 rooms the following year. It was declared a National Historic Landmark in 1987.

Another attraction at Wawona is the Pioneer Yosemite History Center. The center displays several historic buildings that were moved from Yosemite sites, including the Chris Jorgensen Home, George Anderson's Pioneer Home, Hodgdon Homestead Cabin, a blacksmith shop, a cavalry office, a Wells

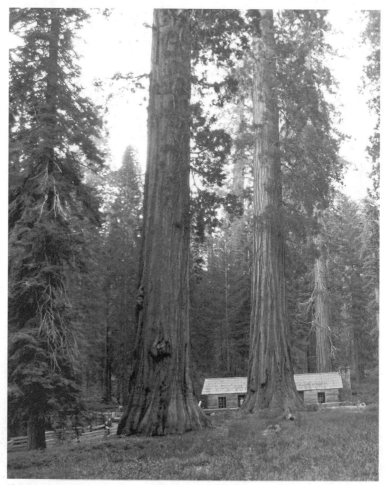

They are huge!

Fargo office, Degnan's Bakery, and a jail. The late ranger Doug Hubbard, chief naturalist at Yosemite 1955–1966, was the driving force behind the project, which opened in 1960.

The main Yosemite Valley lies about an hour north. Another bonus if you arrive via CA 41 (here called the Wawona Road) is that you have access to the connector road to Glacier Point. A diversion to Glacier Point is well worth the extra time. The 13-mile road takes you near California's first ski resort, Badger Pass Ski Resort. Continuing east, you will see a large parking lot at Washburn Point, which reveals the profile of Half Dome. Crowds are smaller here, or you can continue to Glacier Point itself. Facilities include restrooms, a gift shop, and a snack area. The vista point overlooking the entire

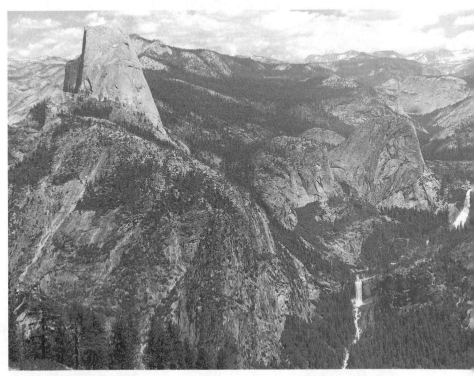

The Giant Staircase

Yosemite Valley is a highlight. From this vantage you can gaze 3,000 feet down on the valley, with clear views of the Giant Staircase showing Vernal and Nevada falls.

The view is often seen in posters of the park, as it encompasses El Capitan, Half Dome, and all the major formations. This perspective of Half Dome reveals that only about 20%

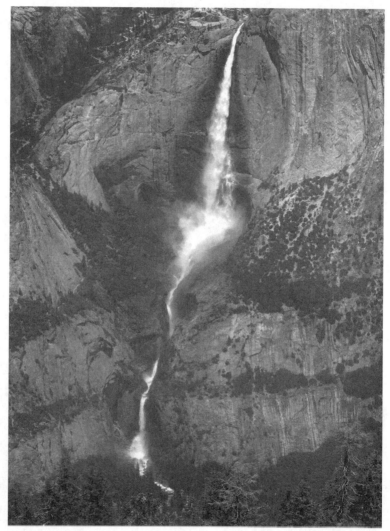

Yosemite Falls from Sentinel Dome

of it is sheared off. Before getting back on the road, you may want to take the short hike to the top of Sentinel Dome; views there are among the best in the park.

Back on the Wawona Road, stop at the left overlook after exiting the long tunnel for another classic valley view.

Finally, you enter the valley proper and can make a quick stop to see Bridalveil Fall up close before arriving at your accommodations. The Mariposa Battalion camped near here in 1851, and John Muir brought President Teddy Roosevelt here for one of their nature talks. Of all the big waterfalls at the park, Bridalveil tends to run longer. The watershed has more soil underlayment, which holds water, while most other falls are in areas of granite, which sheds water sooner. Also, Bridalveil has more of a northern-facing position, so snow does not melt as fast. Be cautious and don't climb on the rocks at the base of the falls.

Arriving via CA 140 Northbound

Southwestern access to the park is from Merced via CA 140. Visitors from central California arrive via this route, which is accessed from CA 99 or I-5. The road from Merced is a gentle, flat road across the farmlands of the Central Valley. The area near Catheys Valley is a notorious CHP speed trap—honor the speed limits. The route also crosses the famous CA 49, which passes many of the old gold-mining sites. If you have time, explore Hornitos, Coulterville, Agua Fria, and the other historic locations. Rolling hills greet you as you enter the historic town of Mariposa, which has an "old west" town ambience. A worthwhile stop is the Mariposa Museum & History Center, which houses many artifacts from the gold-mining days and early Yosemite history. Its coverage of the story of John C. Fremont and his role in early California is excellent.

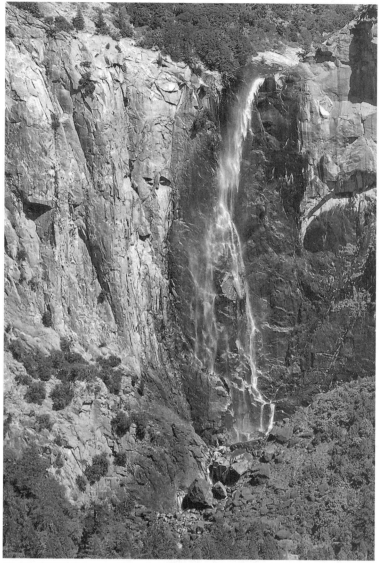

Bridalveil Fall in late summer

Another fun stop is the county courthouse; built in 1854, it's the oldest courthouse west of the Rockies.

After passing Midpines and the Bureau of Land Management information center at Briceburg, you soon arrive at the Ferguson Ridge rockfall. As mentioned earlier, this 2006

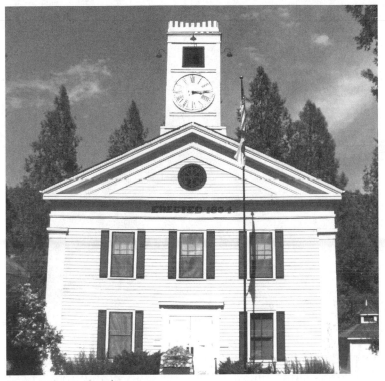

Mariposa County Courthouse

event completely blocked the highway. You may experience delays as one-way traffic is routed from the damaged side of the road, across a one-lane bridge, and then back around the problem. An automated stoplight changes every 15 minutes.

Just a few miles before the park you will pass the small settlement of El Portal. The long-gone Del Portal Hotel housed park visitors arriving by train before they were transferred to carriages (then motor coaches) for transfer to the valley. Many National Park Service employees live in El Portal. The station house and water towers of Bagby were thankfully moved to El Portal when that town was flooded to make way for Lake Don Pedro. Bagby was on the old Merced to Yosemite rail line. A nice display with a locomotive and a caboose is available for

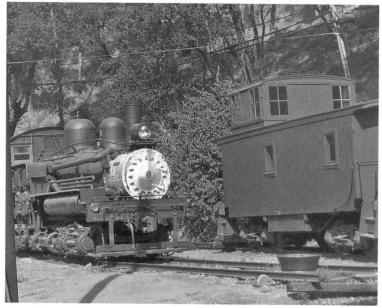

El Portal train display

viewing at the Yosemite Conservancy building in El Portal. The road follows the Merced River Canyon into the park at the Arch Rock entrance. As you approach the park, notice the glaciated canyon walls.

Arriving via CA 120 Westbound

From Nevada, CA 120 brings visitors from Reno, Carson City, and Lake Tahoe via US 395 and the Lee Vining area directly into the northeastern part of the park. Entrance to Yosemite is via the Tioga Pass entrance. However, this road is *not* snowplowed during the winter and often remains inaccessible through at least late May, so plan accordingly. If the pass is closed, the only alternative is to backtrack to I-80 and Sacramento, and then take CA 99 to CA 120 east into the park. Fun stops on US 395 at Mono Lake and the ghost town of Bodie make this route exciting. Once a bustling gold-mining center with 10,000 people, Bodie made many people

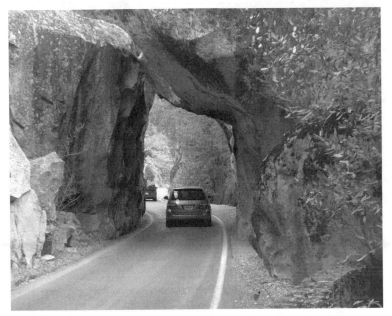

The Arch Rock

rich through the late 1800s and early 1900s. Fires destroyed
most of the original 2,000 wooden buildings, and by 1915 it
was pretty much abandoned. About 50 of the structures still
remain as a California state park with rangers living on-site.
The town is in a state of arrested decay, which means the
buildings are not restored and will be allowed to suffer the
ravaging winters and stifling summers and then vaporize.
Many of the buildings are open for viewing. My favorite is
the schoolhouse, with old-time desks sitting before an old
anatomy chart. It feels almost as though it's recess except for
the layers of dust. Another favorite is the saloon, where you
can see poker tables with chips lined up and bottles of "courage" on shelves. Behind the settlement stands the mine with a
large conveyor belt that was used to process the ore.

Another rewarding side trip is a stop at the remnants of the
Bennettville Silver Mine. It lies about 2 miles east of the
Tioga entrance on national forest land. Look for the Junction

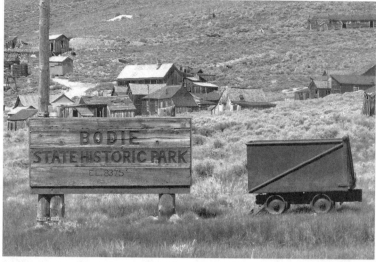

Bodie

Campground on the northeast side of CA 120. An easy trail leads from the parking lot up to the remnants at about 9,900 feet altitude. In the 1880s speculators discovered a silver vein in the hillsides. With investors from New Bedford, Connecticut, bankrolling the operation, the mining town (named for Thomas Bennett Jr., president of the Great Sierra Consolidated Silver Company) sprang up on the hillsides. The projected worker population was 50,000 people. By 1882 8 tons of mining equipment had been shipped to the site. However, no profit was ever made from the mine, despite the use of heavy drilling equipment and a 2,000-foot horizontal shaft. After two years, the investors gave up, and the mine and buildings were abandoned and left to disappear under the brutal Sierra winters. One benefit of this effort was the construction of the Great Sierra Wagon Road, which became the precursor to the Tioga Road, completed in 1961. The mine entrance has been barred so you cannot enter it, but a large tailing field, artifacts, and some old equipment tell the story of what could have been.

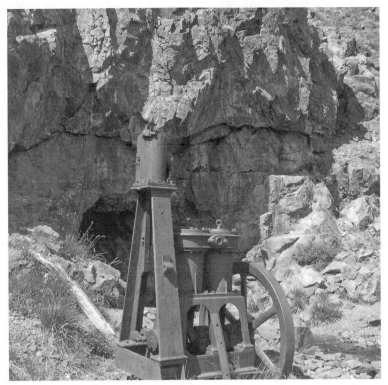

Bennettville mine shaft

Once you enter Yosemite through the Tioga entrance, views of the high peaks are spectacular. Access to Mt. Dana is available near the entrance gate. As you work your way through the high country and toward the valley, you will pass through beautiful Tuolumne Meadows. Be sure to catch the view of Half Dome at Olmsted Point. From this perspective, it looks much different than when viewed from the valley. Here also you can view erratics—large boulders that were carried by the glaciers and gently placed down as they melted. Drive the speed limit, as it's easy to go fast. Many bears are hit each year on the Tioga Road. You will arrive in the valley in about an hour.

Arriving via CA 120 Eastbound

Since the majority of visitors to Yosemite arrive from the west and the greater San Francisco area, I will elaborate on this route. Traveling east on Interstates 580, 205, and 5, you'll soon follow the signs to CA 120 and Yosemite. Upon arriving at Oakdale, you'll see the last significant collection of fast food, gas stations, and strip malls. If you forgot to pack anything, this will be your chance to stock up before entering the park. You should top off your gas tank here. There are a few gas stations before the park, but prices rise dramatically. Be forewarned—*no gas is available in Yosemite Valley.* (However, Crane Flat, just inside the park, does have a gas station.) Also, this may be your last good cell coverage, so make any calls before you head east.

Continuing, you will soon enter the foothills of the Sierra. These are beautiful rolling hills with very rocky soil that discourages the planting of crops. Eight miles east of Oakdale, keep your eyes out on the left side for a memorial to a horse named Cricket. Here you'll see a few wilted wreaths honoring a gray mare that once stood at the fence by the road to watch traffic. Every time I drove the route in the 1990s, Cricket would be patiently waiting to welcome us to her turf. When she died, a small sign with a metal horse figurine on top was erected, and people added flowers and wreaths in her memory. In our fast-paced world, it's nice to know people missed their equine friend. Be careful of traffic if you pull over for a closer look.

As you continue on CA 120, you will come to the little town of Knights Ferry. Turn left down the road to visit a very interesting place. In 1848 Dr. William Knight operated a water taxi to transport gold miners across the Stanislaus River (pronounced "Stan-is-law"). This bargelike system was in effect until a bridge was constructed in 1863. Although beefed up .since

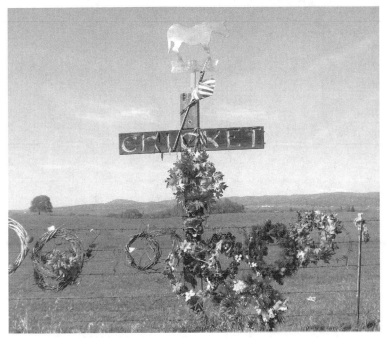

Cricket—gone but not forgotten

its construction, this is one of the oldest and one of the few remaining covered bridges in the western United States. It is the longest covered bridge west of the Mississippi.

Over time, the ferry grounds housed a sawmill, a flour mill, and a power-generating station. At some point a large turbine was installed to provide electricity to the area. Ruins of this complex still exist today. The Army Corps of Engineers operates a visitor center featuring a diorama that describes the role the area played in the dynamic gold rush era. It's well worth stopping at Knights Ferry, which is a cute collection of antiques stores, historic houses, a vintage steel cube jail, and an old-time fire station. If you have time, you can tour the ruins and take a white-water raft trip with one of the many operators in town.

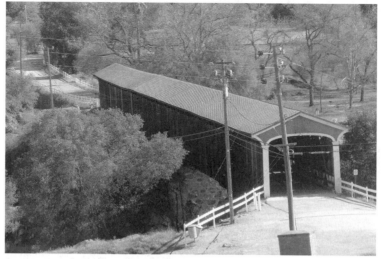

Over the Stanislaus River

Continue on CA 120/108 and be alert for a hard right turn as the road heads east. CA 108 continues straight to Sonora. Watch for the YOSEMITE HWY 120 sign. This general area is known as the Gold Country. The mining towns of Jamestown, Columbia, and others are fun diversions near here. Gold mines in California once produced more than 24 million ounces of the precious metal. Multiply this number by the current gold price and you can understand why California is called the Golden State! There is still plenty of gold in the ground, but environmental concerns make reopening mines difficult. Mercury and cyanide were used to separate gold from other debris—not too healthy. Also, mines of the day ran Pelton waterwheel pumps to remove the underground water, and the mines long ago filled up. A fun and educational detour is up CA 49 to Grass Valley, Nevada City, and the Empire Mine (now a state park). It's the oldest, largest, and richest gold mine in California—5.8 million ounces of gold were pulled out and 367 miles of tunnels and shafts were dug under 5 square miles of that claim.

The next attraction on Highway 120 that you will see is an immense stack of logs that often reaches more than 80 feet high. Raw logs are brought here for processing, and boards are cut in the large mills. This lumber mill is not open for tours, but you will be amazed at the neat stacks, which are equipped with water sprinklers to keep fire danger down. This complex is owned by Sierra Pacific Industries, the third-largest private landowner in the United States. This family-owned business manages 1.5 million acres of California timberlands and produces millwork, lumber, and wood-fiber products.

Just up the road is the very small settlement of Chinese Camp, which was once home to nearly 5,000 Chinese immigrants who worked the gold mines. At its peak, the camp boasted several stores, hotels, joss houses (temples), blacksmiths, a church, a bank, a Wells Fargo office, a Masonic lodge, and a Sons of Temperance building. Few historic structures remain,

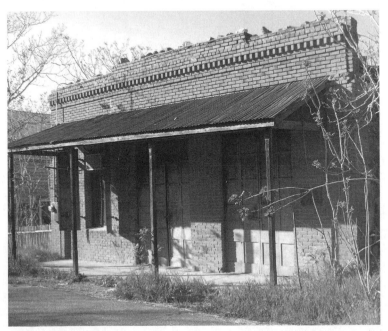

1849 Wells Fargo Office

but a 3-minute drive down Main Street will take you back more than 100 years.

Next you will pass Don Pedro Lake, a man-made reservoir ringed by 160 miles of shoreline and containing nearly 13,000 surface acres of water. It offers a houseboat marina, a boat-launch ramp, fishing, and 172 campsites. The present shoreline of the lake was created in 1971 when the New Don Pedro Dam of the Tuolumne River was completed, replacing a dam built in 1923. The Tuolumne flows out of Yosemite.

Continuing on CA 120 for 5 miles, you will arrive at a very small area known as Moccasin. An interesting fish hatchery is located there and open to the public. Called the Moccasin Creek Hatchery, it is operated by the California Department of Fish and Game and consists of eight large tanks holding fry of varying sizes; a self-serve machine dispenses a handful of feed for you to toss to the fish. These rainbow trout

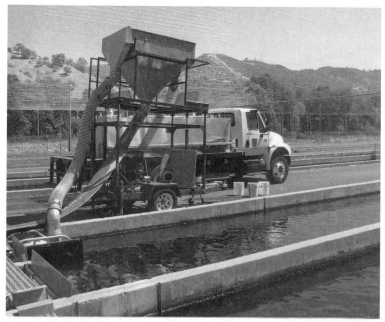

Moccasin Creek Hatchery

THE FIGHT OVER HETCH HETCHY

The melodious name Hetch Hetchy comes from the Native American word for a grass with edible seeds that grows in the area. Following the 1906 earthquake and the severe lack of water that contributed to the raging fires, San Francisco sought a solution. The city appealed to the U.S. Department of the Interior for the water rights to the Tuolumne River in Yosemite. After a 7-year fight by environmentalists (led by John Muir and the Sierra Club), Congress passed the Raker Act, permitting the flooding of the Hetch Hetchy Valley. In 1923 the O'Shaughnessy Dam was completed. As a result of subsequent expansion, it now reaches 430 feet high. The controversy has not ended, with many now advocating the removal of the dam to restore the pristine valley.

are released as part of the state's stocking program. I've seen monsters more than 18 inches long in the tank!

At Moccasin, you can also see the historic power-generating station, a San Francisco Power and Water facility. (It's not open for tours.) In 1921 San Francisco obtained the rights to construct the Hetch Hetchy dam on the Tuolumne River to provide water and electricity to the growing city. At the power station, an engineering marvel built in the Art Deco style, you can see four 12-foot-diameter pipes that carry water over and through the mountains, nearly 200 miles to the San Francisco Bay area reservoirs for distribution. Turbines here provide power from the Moccasin plant.

Immediately after leaving the fish hatchery, you will need to make a choice of roads: to drive the Old Priest Grade or the New Priest Grade. They merge at the top of the hill, so either

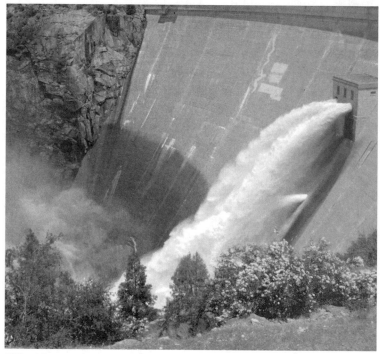

O'Shaughnessy Dam at Hetch Hetchy

will work. Both take you up about 1,575 feet. The winding, steep (17% grade) Old Priest Grade road is the original path that was first a wagon route called Grizzly Gulch Road. It was built in the rush to exploit the park in the 1850s, and it could take a heavy cargo wagon 5 hours to reach the top. Today a strong car engine is limited to 25 mph but can get you up the 2.7 miles in about 10 minutes. If you continue straight on CA 120, you enter the New Priest Grade. This longer road (6 miles) was built in 1915 and is now officially the Priest Grade. It is a saner 4% grade but will slow you down, as tour buses and motor homes wisely take this route. At the top of the grade, both roads converge at Priest's Station. In its heyday it sported a hotel that also served meals to weary travelers, but a huge fire up the gulch in 1926 burned it to the ground. Stop at the top at the newly constructed Priest

Station Cafe & Store to settle your nerves. A deck overlooks Grizzly Gulch. The site still contains the original water well, and an old garage serves as the office. On the return trip, your brakes may smell bad or smoke if you take the Old Priest Grade, so I suggest driving the safer New Priest Grade.

Continuing east on CA 120, you quickly pass through the settlement of Big Oak Flat, which at one time actually featured a very large oak tree. However, in their zest to find gold, miners dug away at the base of the tree, and it later fell. The next town east is Groveland, a fun place to stop for a bite to eat before continuing on. (Groveland's original name was Garrote, coined after a hanging there.) The Iron Door Saloon is California's oldest bar! Groveland also boasts a nice museum with artifacts, photos, and stories from the 1800s. The highway roughly follows the 1874 route into the park.

Entering Yosemite

Regardless of your entry point into the park, you will be greeted by a friendly ranger. Admission is currently $20 per car and is good for a week. An America the Beautiful pass for $80 will gain you admission to any national park and many other federal facilities. A real bargain is the lifetime senior pass. For a one-time fee of only $10, persons over 62 years of age gain admission for themselves and anyone in their vehicle.

Please drive safely. You may not be accustomed to the mountain hairpin turns and limited visibility. Pass cautiously. Much of your travel will be on two-lane roads with sharp cliffs just feet away. If you are slower than the flow of traffic, use a turnout to let others by. Do not speed; speed limits are enforced throughout the park.

Lastly, please consider taking public transportation to the park. The Yosemite Area Rapid Transit System (YARTS) provides service from outlying communities and also over the Tioga Road into Mammoth Lakes during the summer season. Gear, including bicycles and hiking equipment, can be brought on any YARTS bus. All fares to Yosemite include gate fees. Bus service between Yosemite Valley and El Portal is very reasonable, with kids under age 12 getting a discount. Senior discounts and family packages are also available. Many park employees use YARTS, so you may get a chance to talk to a ranger. Once inside the valley, the free hybrid-powered shuttle bus system can get you to most attractions.

The official address for the park is:

Superintendent
Yosemite National Park
9039 Village Drive
P.O. Box 577
Yosemite, CA 95389
(209) 372-0201

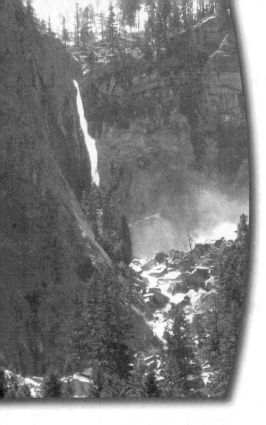

7
Preparation

*The mountains are calling and
I must go.*

—John Muir

Preparation is the key to any successful undertaking. I suggest you plan your trip several months in advance. Your three "critical path" elements are: (1) accommodations, (2) permits, and (3) conditioning. You'll need enough time to secure a place to stay. You'll also need time to gradually get in shape, get your equipment, break it in, and take several practice hikes.

Accommodations

There are many alternatives for rooms in and near Yosemite. Keep in mind how popular the park is (4 million visitors a year) and that many will be competing with you for rooms. Call very early in your planning process; you can always cancel within a week of arrival. Web-based companies, travel agents, and AAA are all good sources to consult. Depending on your needs, you can secure a motel room, a cabin, or a tent site. Due to the magnitude of the Half Dome hike, I highly recommend in-park Yosemite Valley accommodations. You will need to be well rested for the hike and will want to eat and sleep soon after your hike. Off-park sites will add almost an hour to both ends of the hike. The park concessionaire, Delaware North Companies Parks & Resorts at Yosemite, Inc. (DNC), currently operates a number of lodging facilities in Yosemite National Park under contract with the National Park Service, and they provide many accommodation options. Most can be reserved up to a year and a day in advance. I suggest you call the minute they open. You're competing with much of the nation (and foreign visitors as well) for the dates you want. You will be charged for the first night, but it is refundable if you cancel before seven days of your arrival. It is worth the investment to ensure you get a place. Reservations for all Yosemite overnight accommodations can be obtained by phone at (801) 559-5000 (DNC) for lodging and (800) 436-7275 (**recreation.gov**) for camping. If things are fully booked and you are patient, you may also secure a place when cancellations come in. The park website has excellent descriptions of all facilities; see **yosemitepark.com.**

CURRY VILLAGE

Curry Village has a long and hallowed history from when it was first known as Camp Sequoia, then Camp Curry. Opened in 1899 by David and Jenny Curry, it was designed as a cheap lodging option for valley visitors. Located at the east end of the valley, it is a gateway to many of the park's eastern attractions. The horse stables, Vernal and Nevada falls, the John Muir Trail, Half Dome, and Glacier Point are all accessible from Curry Village without driving through the park. Today it offers a variety of lodging options, including 18 standard motel rooms, 100 cabins with private baths, 3 specialty cabins with baths, 80 cabins with central bathhouses, and 427 canvas tent cabins. Curry Village boasts a grocery and gift store, eateries, an outdoor pool, bicycle and raft rentals, children's programs, a comprehensive tour/activity desk, and a mountaineering school and mountain shop.

If you are not staying in the Curry Village area, you will need to get there to be near the trailhead. There is a large backpacker parking lot just east of Curry for your use.

TENT CABINS

My recommended accommodations for your adventure are the Curry Village tent cabins. These shelters have wood frames and floors and white canvas tops and sides. They sleep up to four people and are equipped with spring beds, bedding, towels, and a small safe. Each has a single lightbulb (no outlets) and a wooden door with a padlock. No cooking is permitted in or near the tent cabins. Shared toilets are nearby. Men's and women's shower facilities are located in the central part of the village, and their use is included with

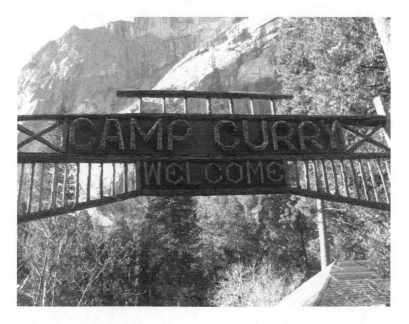

your reservation. The showers get crowded 4–6 p.m. as day hikers return to camp. Lines may be long, but the hot water is plentiful. Bring sandals, soap, and shampoo. Rates for tent cabins are less than typical motel prices. Be sure to check for current prices.

WOOD CABINS

The wood cabins are much more substantial and comfortable than the tent cabins. For visitors who prefer a little more privacy, the wood cabins can satisfy this and also provide a more rustic mood. They are in the same general area as the other Curry Village accommodations, with easy access to nearby services.

FIREFALL

One very interesting event once held at Camp Curry was the nightly Firefall. From its initiation in 1872, at 9 p.m. each summer night, workers above the camp at Glacier Point would begin to push burning embers over the edge to cascade down toward the rocks behind Camp Curry in an orchestrated display. The spectacle resembled a waterfall of fire. Some who saw the spectacle when they were children have told me that it was surreal, and that the glowing embers cascading down the granite looked like something from a fairy tale. The Firefalls were stopped in January 1968, when the park service decided that this show was not in keeping with the mission of the organization. The meadows were being trampled by hordes of spectators, and thefts increased during show hours. You can briefly see the Firefall in action in the 1954 movie *The Caine Mutiny*.

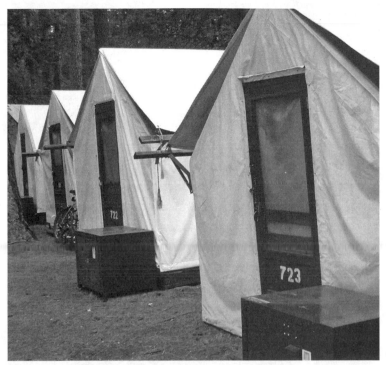

Tent cabins offer economical accommodations.

TENT CAMPING

Yosemite has 13 excellent campgrounds, and most are reservable. Three sites in the eastern Yosemite Valley are convenient to the hike. They are North, Upper, and Lower Pines. Another, Camp 4, is farther away and is first come, first served. It is on the National Register of Historic Places because of its role in big-wall climbing, and many climbers stay there. The Pines offer about 400 spots and are economical. Depending on your budget and ability to sleep soundly on the ground, tent camping may be for you. These sites may be reserved up to five months in advance. Reservations can be made by calling the National Park Reservation System at (800) 436-7275 or online at **recreation.gov.** Be sure to follow bear-safe storage of your food and any scented items (toothpaste, cologne, and so on). See the Bears section in Chapter 5, Precautions.

HOUSEKEEPING CAMP

The Housekeeping Camp, which is a step above traditional dirt camping, is located along the Merced River. Its location is also a good kick-off point for the Half Dome hike. The complex consists of 266 units, each holding up to six people. Structurally, there are three concrete walls, with the entrance being a sliding curtain. Each unit has two single bunk beds, a double bed, a table, chairs, a mirror, electrical lights, and outlets. You must bring your own linens or sleeping bag. Housekeeping Camp's lodging does not include housekeeping service, despite the odd name. A handy Laundromat is located nearby. Restroom facilities here are communal.

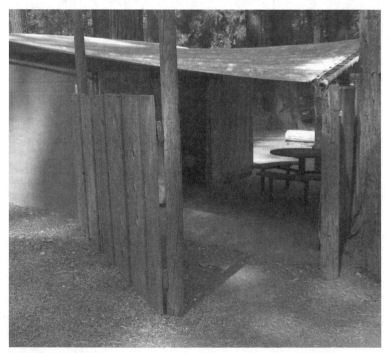

Housekeeping Camp

IN-PARK MOTELS AND HOTELS

Yosemite Lodge at the Falls is a nice vintage motel in the center of the valley. It was upgraded in 1998, and the units are comfortable and clean. This is a nice, central location, offering 226 lodge rooms, 19 standard rooms, and 4 family rooms. Reserve by phone at (559) 253-5635.

The ultimate luxury is the Ahwahnee Hotel. Opened in 1927, the Ahwahnee is on par with fine hotels in any major city and has hosted presidents and world leaders. It has 123 rooms, consisting of 99 hotel rooms (with parlors and suites) and 24 cottages. One summer, my hiking party failed to secure other lodging, so we split the cost of an Ahwahnee room—a wonderful luxury for weary hikers at the end of the day.

Many other fine accommodations are available in Yosemite, but they are too far from the trailhead for Half Dome to be

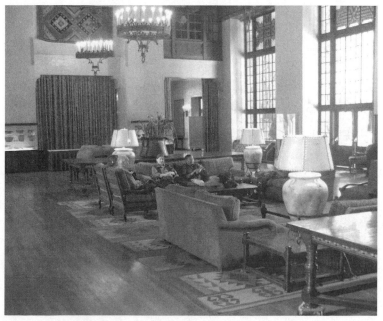

Inside the Ahwahnee Hotel

practical. Tuolumne Meadows Lodge, Wawona Hotel, and White Wolf Lodge should all be considered for your future trips to other destinations in the park. Rental lodging at Foresta and Yosemite West may also interest you. They are on private land grandfathered before the area was part of the park.

ACCOMMODATIONS OUTSIDE THE PARK

Motels to the east of the park are not advised since they are too far from the valley for this hike, and CA 120 might be closed with snow over Tioga Pass early in the summer. All three western access routes to the park are loaded with motels. CA 120, CA 140, and CA 41 are all home to many types of dwellings, from large complexes to quaint lodges. The only problem with staying outside the park is the long drive to the trailhead. It is more than 40 minutes from most western entrance gates to the valley floor, so you'll need to add that to your time. It's not a fun drive to do when you're dead tired after a very long hike.

INTERNET

In this day of personal connection it's nice to know that the park does provide access to the World Wide Web. At Curry Village you can connect at the Curry Lounge. Demand is high, so access can be difficult. Free Wi-Fi is provided; bring your laptop. Do not download photos, videos, or use VOIP (voice over internet protocol). They bog down the bandwidth and degrade performance for everyone. At the Yosemite Lodge, access is free if you are staying there or for a small fee if you drop in. At the Ahwahnee Hotel, access is also free for guests. Visitors can also access the Web at the Valley Library, but I find it too far off, and its hours are limited. There are thoughts of providing Internet access to the entire valley.

Permits

Since 2010, permits have been required every day of the week for all visitors who want to hike to the top of Half Dome. It applies 24/7. The process described here is current as of publication. Yosemite is developing a long-term plan for the use of the Half Dome trail and cables called the Half Dome Stewardship Plan. The final approved document may alter these procedures. Please refer to the park's website for the latest information: **nps.gov/yose/planyourvisit/hdpermits.htm.** I will also post all regulations about Half Dome on my website/blog: **hikehalfdome.com.**

Everyone must carry a permit to go beyond Sub Dome, the 400-foot granite hill just before the cables. Half Dome bigwall climbers may come up the face and down the cables without a permit. Protection division rangers at Sub Dome will check permits and enforce the permit requirement. A maximum of 400 hikers will be allowed (300 day hikers and 100 backpackers with a wilderness permit) each day on the Half Dome trail beyond Sub Dome. These numbers may be changed in the future.

HOW TO APPLY FOR A PERMIT

Permits will be distributed by lottery via **recreation.gov.** You must apply March 1–31 for all trips when the cables are up. Go to **recreation.gov** or call (877) 444-6777 (call center is open 7 a.m.–9 p.m. PST; online requests can be made anytime during a lottery period).

On each application, you can apply for up to six permits (six people) and for up to seven dates. Applications will only be successful if the number of permits requested is available on at least one of the requested dates. If enough permits are available for more than one of the requested dates, permits will be automatically awarded to the highest priority date, as entered by the applicant. Applicants may apply as the trip leader only once per lottery and must specify their name; applicants may specify the name of an alternate trip leader as well. Multiple applications with the same trip leader will be removed from the lottery, and any person applying multiple times as trip leader will have their lottery applications canceled. Permits will only be valid if the trip leader and/or alternate specified on the permit is part of the group using the permits. The names of the trip leader and alternate may not be changed once the application is submitted, and the permits are not transferable.

PRESEASON LOTTERY

Permits for the hiking season will be distributed by lottery in early April. Applicants will receive an e-mail notification of lottery results in early April (or can get results online or by calling **recreation.gov**).

DAILY LOTTERY

In addition, 50 permits will be available each day by lottery during the hiking season. These permits will be available based on the estimated rate of under-use and cancellation of permits (the exact number may change through the summer). Daily lotteries will have an application period two days prior to the hiking date with a notification late that night. (Example: To hike on Saturday, you would apply on Thursday morning and receive an e-mail notification of results late Thursday night. Results will also be available online or by phone the next morning.) The application period will be midnight–1 p.m. PST.

FEES

Two separate fees are collected. The first fee, which is charged at the time you submit an application, is $4.50 (online) or $6.50 (by phone). This nonrefundable fee, which is per application (not per person), is charged by **recreation.gov** for the costs of processing your permit application.

The second fee is $5 per person and is charged only when you receive a permit. (This fee also applies to wilderness permit holders.) The $5 fee is fully refundable if you cancel your permit more than two days before the hiking date specified on your permit or if the cables are not up on the date for which your permit is valid.

WILDERNESS PERMITS

People with wilderness permits that reasonably include Half Dome as part of their itinerary will also receive Half Dome permits upon request and without further competition. (Wilderness permits are subject to a quota system.)

Note: This process is very important to understand. To repeat, for the latest updates go to **nps.gov/yose/planyourvisit/ hdpermits.htm** and **hikehalfdome.com.**

Conditioning

I suggest you begin your serious Half Dome training about two months prior to your trip. This, of course, depends on what regime you now follow (at least 30 minutes of exercise per day is recommended by doctors). Advance training will allow you to build the muscle and endurance required. By starting your conditioning early, you will have time to recover from any injury prior to the hike. To successfully get to the top and not feel like a dishrag afterward, being in shape is critical. True, you might be able to just jump out of the car with no preparation and do the hike, but you'll regret it. The day after my first hike up Half Dome, my quads were so sore that it felt better to walk backwards! If you haven't had a physical exam in a few years, get one. Make sure your doctor gives you the green light for the hike. You'll be doing a lot of stretching, twisting, pulling, and movements that you may not be accustomed to. If you have asthma, get your doctor's ok. Be sure to bring your inhaler. If you are middle-aged or older (or young and curious), you may want to get a treadmill stress test. Medical personnel hook you up to electrodes and put you on a moving treadmill that gets faster and steeper every 2 minutes. Doctors are present to monitor your heart rhythm and your ability to reach a heart rate close to your calculated maximum. They also monitor your ability to return to your resting heart rate in a prescribed time.

Start your training by walking 30–45 consecutive minutes. Build your sessions until you can walk well over an hour at a good pace. Try to walk as if you're crossing a street with the WALK sign blinking (that is, walk briskly). If you are able to jog, progress to running 2–3 miles at a moderate pace (10–11 minutes per mile). We're trying to build up endurance. Find some hills and move your workouts there. Running uphill is great, but walk downhill to protect your knees. Throw in some biking too; it's great for the legs. If you can get to a gym, a stair stepper will be your best friend. For what you'll be doing on your hike, it will give the best return on your investment. However, I prefer reality to gym equipment, and a stair stepper does nothing for your downhill muscles. Your shins will hurt if you train only for uphills. If you live in a flat area of the country, find a tall building and walk the fire escape stairs. Cross-training with elliptical trainers, stationary bikes, and a good step aerobics class will all help. The rowing machine is one of the best overall workouts you can get, and Nordic Walking is a fun fitness activity that will improve your stamina. Build up endurance and calluses (you don't want to experience blisters on the hike).

Do a lot of training hikes. Your Half Dome hike will be about 16 miles plus a mile up and down. Build up to this number on your training hikes. Also, you should be gauging your water and food needs so you are not surprised on the actual hike.

You will need upper body strength to get up the cables, so you also need to focus there. Biceps curls, triceps work, chest pulls, and so on will pay off. If you do not know how to properly lift weights, talk to a personal trainer. Always start out with lighter weights to avoid injury. Try to do 8–10 reps with three sets.

When you're within a month of the trip, seek out some nice long hills to hike on. The steeper, the better. I really believe that the best way to get in shape for an activity is to *do* the activity. Hike, hike, hike. Work up to 90 minutes, then 3 hours, and ultimately about 6 hours. By the time you can hike about 6 hours, you should be enjoying yourself and looking forward to the Half Dome adventure. Take the last few hikes with all the gear you'll be bringing to Yosemite. You should wear your boots as much as possible to get them broken in. On hike day you may be walking for 12–13 hours—can you do that during your training?

Remember to stretch after every workout. Hold each pose for about 20 seconds and don't bounce. The three major areas to stretch are your quads, calves, and hamstrings.

In the last week, taper down; do nothing before the hike. You need to rest up, and you don't want any injuries. Stressing your body close to your hike day could negatively impact you.

What to Bring

This will be a simple, time-tested list. It's what I bring. Modify it to your preferences and budget; whatever works for you is perfect. I'll discuss what to bring in the order of importance. The categories are water, food, clothes, and other gear essentials.

WATER

Water is the most important factor on this hike. You do not want to skimp on drinking. Dehydration will sap your energy and cause you to think irrationally. It can also have severe medical consequences. Your choices are to bring all the water you'll need or to treat the water along the trail.

With the first alternative, you'll need to haul up a *lot* of water. How much should you bring? I weigh about 200 pounds and drink 7 quarts in the course of the day. I don't like this alternative because water is heavy—about 2 pounds per quart. Why carry this extra weight for all those miles? And how do you carry it? In a backpack this weight would really cut into your shoulders, and your back would be soaked with sweat. The bladder-type backpack systems are popular, but I don't like them because they add a lot of weight on your back and can carry only a limited amount of water. The biggest bladder I've seen only holds 3 quarts. After several hours, your lower back may begin to ache. When you carry all your water, it will get warm from your body and the atmosphere. Another major concern is that you will begin to ration your water by sipping instead of hydrating. Two thumbs up for alternative two: treat the water.

In addition to the issue of *having* water is the problem of removing impurities. The three major types of pathogenic microorganisms and their sizes are:

1. Protozoans: amebiasis, *Giardia lamblia, Cryptosporidium:* 1–15 microns

2. Bacteria: E. coli, salmonella, cholera: 0.2–5 microns

3. Viruses: hepatitis A, Norwalk virus, rotavirus, poliovirus: 0.02–0.2 microns

These can be negated chemically, mechanically, or with ultraviolet light. (Boiling is not feasible unless you are camping.)

Chemical Treatment Since World War I we have used iodine to treat water. The iodine kills many, but not all, of the most common pathogens present in natural freshwater sources. A major drawback at Yosemite is that iodine is not effective against *Cryptosporidium.* It does have medium effectiveness on giardia and a high effectiveness on bacteria and viruses. Iodine can be extremely dangerous if used in incorrect quantities, if used over an extended period of time (more than a few weeks), or if the hiker is pregnant or has a thyroid disease. This could lead to serious hyperthyroidism. Iodine-based tablets have a usable open bottle life of only three months. The Centers for Disease Control recommends against using iodine as your main water purification/treatment method on a multiweek long-distance backpacking trip. In fact, the European Union has banned the sale of iodine water purification drops and tablets. That aside, the way iodine or other chemical products work is to place a tablet into the water, and then wait 30 minutes for it to do its thing. The process takes longer for cold or turbid water. Another major downside to this method is that you will have to sit at the water source while the chemical action takes place. Then you will be drinking an iodine-flavored mixture; however, taste-neutralizing tablets can be used to mellow out the foul taste. If you want more water, you will have to wait another 30-minute period. When you are hiking Half Dome, you need to be drinking constantly, and the wait period will slow you down. Other possible chemicals that can be used to treat water include chlorine, chlorine dioxide, and sodium hypochlorite (bleach). These can be harmful, so use caution.

Mechanical Treatment A high-quality mechanical water treatment pump makes this chore easy and isn't very expensive. The three types of mechanical devices to treat water, their functions, and their micron ratings are:

Filter (1–4 microns): Removes giardia, large protozoans, and some bacteria.

Microfilter (.3–1 micron): Removes microorganisms, including protozoans and bacteria.

Purifier (<.018 micron): Removes microorganisms, including viruses.

Read the filter's box carefully. The nomenclature can be confusing. The street name for these devices is water filter. However, as you can see above, the technical name implies distinct capabilities. Filters can remove bacteria and protozoan cysts; purifiers can do this *and* remove viruses. (Viruses are not present in most American water sources.) The U.S. Environmental Protection Agency (EPA) requires that a device labeled as a purifier remove viruses (with a rigorous EPA documentation procedure). Be sure to read the literature to make sure if giardia, *Cryptosporidium,* and other microscopic pathogens (disease-causing agents) will be removed. Giardia will be your biggest concern in Yosemite. A 0.3-micron pore size or less is regarded as the optimum. There are many filter brands to choose from, and the sales staff at your outfitter can help you sort this out. A good unit will be lightweight and compact. Many come with a pleated cartridge filter and a bottle adapter. You should be able to pump 1 quart per minute. The life of a cartridge depends on the quality of water you're trying to filter. The cleaner the source, the longer the filter will last. Still water

is better than mov-
ing water because
sediments tend to
sink rather than cir-
culate as they do in
moving water.

You will have a
choice of several
models from vari-
ous manufacturers.

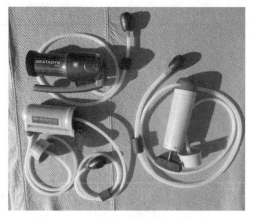

Water filter pumps

Some models have
a piston-type pump mechanism, and others use a lever. Some
have outlets that clip directly into the standard-size wide-
mouth water bottle; some have a small container of granulated
charcoal near the outlet that improves taste. Higher-priced
models are light and pack small. To clean your filter pump, I
suggest cutting a large hole in the top of a half-gallon plastic
milk container. Fill it with tap water and add a capful of household bleach. Then put your inlet and outlet into the water and
circulate-pump it for about 5 minutes. This will flush the system with diluted bleach to kill any hitchhiking bacteria. I also
bring a small zip-top bag to store the clean end of the system, so
I don't get it contaminated by the wet, dirty stream water while
carrying the filter. If your filter is clogged, it will take longer
to pump the water (a sign that cleaning is needed). Follow the
manufacturer's instructions on how to place the intake in the
stream. You'll be amazed at the great job these devices can do
with a small water source. Filters will be effective for about 200
gallons, provided you don't pump water loaded with sediment.

Ultraviolet Light   A relatively new technology for portable
water treatment is the use of ultraviolet (UV) light. UV technology has been used for decades by many cities in their
municipal water treatment plants. When exposed to the

proper wavelength, the DNA of the microbes is affected such that they cannot reproduce. Without reproduction capabilities, the microbes can't make you ill. A company called Hydro-Photon introduced the portable UV water purifier with the brand name SteriPEN. It markets several models that can destroy more than 99.9% of bacteria, viruses, and protozoans. These UV purifiers are effective and battery powered. Water treated by UV technology needs to be as clear as possible to prevent pathogens from hiding behind sediment. It's best to agitate the water during the treatment. The optimum method for unclear water is to first filter it, thereby removing the particulates, prior to using UV purification.

Electrolytes It takes about 4–6 hours for your body to deplete its reserves of essential minerals and electrolytes, so this is one hike for which you should ingest some sort of energy product. Dehydration will ruin your day. You may hit the wall, have poor judgment, and be unable to continue the hike. A good-tasting fluid will encourage you to drink more often. Choosing which product you use will take some experimentation during your training period. Most are easy to carry, and I put my powdered electrolyte crystals in a double zip-top bag to prevent loss. Then I add the product to my freshly treated water, about 2 tablespoons of powdered energy drink mix per quart. Since I carry two 1-quart bottles,

A quart is almost the same volume as a liter. There are 32 ounces in a quart and 34 ounces in a liter. I talk about them interchangeably. A quart of water weighs 2 pounds. I have kept track of my water needs, and I drink 7 quarts on the all-day Half Dome hike. If I carried that much water, it would weigh 14 pounds—a very large weight to haul for 16 miles. Your training hikes will help you find what your body needs.

I try to keep a balance of one bottle of clear water and one bottle of energy drink.

Dehydration impairs human performance whenever the body's fluid level falls below 98% of normal. The main cause of dehydration is fluid loss through sweating. Sweating is a good process, since it releases heat generated by working muscles to the air. It is the body's cooling mechanism. It has been known for decades that the performance of athletes is hampered by a loss of fluids, electrolytes, and carbohydrates. Dehydration strains the cardiovascular system by reducing blood volume. For every liter of fluid lost during prolonged exercise, body temperature rises by 0.3°C, heart rate elevates by about eight beats per minute, and the volume of blood pumped by the heart per minute declines by 1 liter per minute.

Drink before you're thirsty is a great guideline. Your practice hikes will show you how much water you need. The old sailor's rule is that you should pee clear. If you're voiding yellow, you perhaps are *not* drinking enough.

Water Bottles Canteen-type containers and small-mouth bottles are awkward on the trail and are very hard to refill. I prefer to take two 1-quart, wide-mouthed hard plastic camping bottles. The better models have an attached screw top and are virtually indestructible. Most have taken the questionable chemical BPA out of their production process. They're leak-proof and can be dropped without fear of their breaking. Their wide mouth provides for a quick connection to many water-treatment devices. Colored versions provide a quick way to distinguish your bottle from those of your hiking mates. I even use mine as a pillow when resting!

FOOD

The most important meal of the hike is actually the meal you had the night before. The nutrients you consume will take about 12 hours to be digested and fill your energy stores. Eat smart here and don't overdo it. Avoid any foods you are not used to. An emphasis on carbohydrates is advised because this is what your body uses first for fuel. But remember that the carbohydrates you eat the night before may be gone by hike time, so it's safest to balance protein, fat, and carbs and avoid anything that might cause indigestion. The Curry Village Pavilion serves an all-you-can-eat meal. Don't drink alcohol until after your hike; it will actually dehydrate you. You'll be better off sticking to juices. Also, keep caffeine consumption down.

Breakfast on the day of your hike will, by necessity, be abbreviated. Since nothing is open early enough for a sit-down meal, you'll need to bring your own food or stock up at the Curry Village store. Bagels, muffins, fruit, granola, trail mix, and orange juice are all available. Don't overdo it. Be sure to store your food in the metal bear boxes provided.

While on the hike, you can bring a variety of foods, but lean to the carb side. You don't want to deplete your glycogen stores; the resulting fatigue will ruin your day. Avoid anything greasy or fatty. My own experiments have led me to bring seven energy bars, a bag of trail mix, a bag of beef jerky, and some hard candy. The candy will provide sugar and keep your throat moist. Energy bars help deliver carbohydrates to your muscles, brain, and body systems to keep you alert and strong. Most other things will get smashed in your pack. Sandwiches will get squished. The important element is the water you'll be drinking. You don't want to bonk halfway through the hike.

Be a good citizen and pack out all your trash. There are *no* trash cans along the entire route, so you must take out what you bring in. Also, don't toss apple cores or banana peels into the woods. Yes, they are biodegradable, but how long will it take? They will attract ants, bees, and other animals. Let's keep Yosemite beautiful! Have everyone in your party pick up at least one piece of trash on the hike.

Elimination While on the subject of food, we need to address your restroom needs. I suggest you take care of this before you begin your hike, but if not, don't worry. Once on the hike, you will be able to use a nice flushing toilet at the Vernal Fall footbridge. As you continue on, there are three composting toilets; I will point them out when I discuss the actual trail. Since you will be hydrating, you will need to urinate. When you are beyond the last facility at Little Yosemite Valley, you will need to go in the woods. Here is the process: walk at least 100 feet from the trail or any water and urinate on plants. If you go on rocks, the odor will linger. If you need to defecate, you must dig a 6-inch deep cathole. Do your thing and then cover the hole with dirt. In all cases, you are to pack out any toilet paper; bring along a zip-top bag for this. Do not bury the paper, as the weather will expose it. Do not burn it— many forest fires have been started that way. Please follow this procedure. The unpleasant alternative would be human waste disposal kits, which are used in many other parks.

CLOTHES

The general rule for hiking and backpacking is to wear no cotton. This natural fabric absorbs your sweat, rain, and waterfall spray and will not dry rapidly. You will feel clammy as the day wears on. Synthetic fabrics such as polypropylene or nylon derivatives are best. They do not retain moisture and will help you avoid windchill if an afternoon breeze comes up. Think synthetic from top to bottom. Wool blends are also good, but again no cotton.

Shirt   I prefer a long-sleeved polypropylene shirt. The day may start out chilly in the morning, but the summer sun will soon make it pleasant. You can keep your sleeves down in the early morning and fold them up as the day goes on or keep them down for sun protection. A collar will protect your neck from the intense sun later in the day. The standard button-front shirt allows you to open it up for quick cooling. What you wear depends a lot on when you go. June and October trips can be very cold at 6 a.m. The problem is that you must carry everything with you. If you bring a fleece coat to keep warm in the morning, you may end up carrying it the rest of the day. If you hide it for pickup on your return, it may be stolen or viewed as trash and discarded. T-shirts are tempting, but they provide no warmth in the early morning and will be soaked with sweat within a few hours. Also, a long-sleeved shirt provides a pocket or two to hold your energy bar or small camera. Many days it is windy and brisk on Half Dome, so a long-sleeved shirt is handy for cutting the chill.

Pants/Shorts   Lightweight hiking pants or shorts are great for the Half Dome hike. I really like cargo pants with zip-off legs. When it is chilly in the morning, I keep them fastened but can remove them with the heat of the day and store the legs in my pack. I put some trail mix in my large pocket so I don't have to remove my pack to get something to eat. Loose shorts allow you to move freely and should be made of polypropylene or nylon. You don't need heavy-weight hiking shorts. Chafing can be a problem, so you may want to use a lubricating gel on your inner thighs.

Shoes   Your boots are where the rubber meets the road, so to speak. Of all your equipment, nothing is more critical. If you take the time (and spend the money) to get a well-fitting, well-made pair of hiking boots, you'll be far along the way to completing this hike with little pain. High-quality boots (and socks) will keep your feet dry and blister free. The time you spend walking around the shoe store will pay off later. When trying on boots, bring the socks you will be wearing while hiking. Get ankle-high hiking boots. On the Half Dome trail, you'll be walking over many hard granite steps, and stability is important to prevent foot stress and sprains. Your shoes are the heart of your hiking "machine." Depending on your interest in continuing hiking, you may want stretch your budget and buy a pair that will also be good for hiking with a heavy pack.

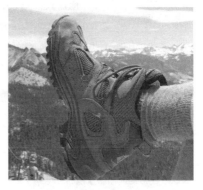

High-quality hiking boots are best.

Don't attempt the hike in smooth-soled or tennis shoes. Repeat: *No tennis shoes*. Why? They're comfortable, aren't they? True, but they're very dangerous on slick rocks. You'll get little traction on the incline of Half Dome. The route up the cables is worn smooth from almost 100 years of use. Modern boots have "snow tire treads" that will allow you to grip the granite confidently. In addition, you'll be stepping on a lot of sharp rocks during the day, and gradually, the feel of those points will go right through to your feet. If your feet get fatigued, this will contribute to a general body fatigue. Also, tennis shoes and econo boots offer little ankle support. A name-brand pair of lightweight hiking boots is recommended. You don't need expedition quality, but you'll be much happier investing in good shoes. They'll last for years, and you can amortize the cost over many seasons of hiking.

Look for water-repellent or Gore-Tex uppers; they will keep your feet dry when crossing streams or in heavy downpours. The shank of the boot is the inner foundation that lies under your foot. Shanks come in many types. The steel shank is popular, offering protection to your sole and arch, but steel is subject to corrosion if you have not sealed your boots properly. Nylon and fiberglass shanks won't rust and are not as sensitive to temperature extremes as steel, and, as an added benefit, they are lighter than steel. Nylon and fiberglass are typically found in higher-priced boots. At the bottom of the line is the fiberboard shank. As you can guess, they're found in very low-end boots and are not recommended.

In recent years, Vibram has become the standard sole for shock protection and long wear. The sole was designed to provide excellent traction on the widest range of surfaces, with a high degree of abrasion resistance. With every season, new shoe materials are being introduced. Cosmetic features, such as leather and nylon mesh, allow for a stylish look. We haven't even talked about welts, midsoles, heel counters, or lacing systems. Here is one time I trust the salesperson. Concentrate on the fit and take your time when shopping. Most good outfitters should have an inclined board to simulate downhill walking. Remember that the second half of the hike is downhill and allow for room in the toe box so your toes don't bang against the end. If the fit is too tight, you could end up with black toenails, or even worse, your nails could fall off. You may want to remove the thin cardboard inner sole your boots come with and put in a foam insole. As you can see, shopping for a good pair of boots can be overwhelming.

Buy boots early and break them in. Take care of your boots, and they will last a long time. Be sure to seal them with the proper treatment chemicals if they are leather. Clean any mud and dirt off them before storing them and keep them in a cool, dry place to prevent mildew from setting in. Take the insole out and check your laces occasionally.

I've seen many people in tennis shoes and even a few in sandals, but I saw it all when I came across a woman doing the hike barefoot with duct tape wrapped over the balls of her feet. No kidding. I don't know if her boyfriend had her shoes in his pack, but this was a first.

Socks   I suggest that you apply an anti-chafing product over your feet to lubricate them. Commercial products are available at outfitters and running stores. Use a thin wicking silk inner sock with a medium-weight hiking sock. This will reduce friction and the chances of a blister. Use this same sock combination when you try on your boots, prior to buying them. You'll be much happier if you buy several pairs of the same socks so that you can rotate them. "Real" hiking socks from your equipment outfitter are recommended. Stay away from using that old pair of basketball socks or tube socks. Hiking socks are engineered (yes, even socks) to provide comfort, sweat wicking, and attention to typical foot hot spots. Keeping your feet dry is the key to avoiding blisters. I like to bring spare socks in my pack and routinely change socks on the summit for the long hike down. Bringing a spare pair will also be useful if your primary pair gets wet on the Mist Trail.

Hat   Much of the hike is in tree shade, but in the last hours to the summit you will be vulnerable to harmful UV rays, so a sun hat is another clothing item that you'll appreciate. Although the hike is balanced between sun and shade, the midday sun can be taxing in the thin air. A wide-brim hat is very functional, but a baseball hat is adequate and can be quickly tucked into your waist when you want to cool off your head a bit. You may consider bringing a clip device that secures your cap to your collar to prevent a strong breeze from pulling your hat off. Soaking your hat with water will bring relief on a hot day.

OTHER ESSENTIALS

Pack   You'll need a container to carry all your necessities. Many hikers like to use a backpack with an integral water bladder. I prefer to do the hike using a fanny pack. My back sweats a lot, and backpacks trap the heat on me. Also, with a large pack, you tend to load up extraneous items that just add weight, which can cause lower back pain. The fanny pack rides at my center of gravity and keeps my back free. It should have large pouches for your water bottles and a small central pouch for food and supplies. Make sure you get a pack that can carry two 1-quart plastic water bottles. (Do not use the smaller bicycle bottles. You'll need all the water you can get.) I bring my water pump to refill along the trail. The fanny pack will allow you to easily remove your bottles from their holster while you are on the move.

Blister Pack   Most outfitters and drugstores will have a selection of blister-preventative products. These are friction-resisting pads, which are best if applied before you get a blister. Once a blister surfaces, you go into mitigation mode. Moleskin is great for isolating the blister from further damage. I also carry a small tube of antiseptic ointment, just in case.

Facecloth   I find that I'm sweating heavily by the time I'm halfway up the Mist Trail. Relying on a shirt sleeve for wiping off sweat doesn't seem to work. I like to carry a small white cotton facecloth, which I simply loop under my fanny pack belt so it dries as I walk. A bonus is that if you keep a corner of it clean, it's great for cleaning your glasses.

Sunglasses   Stark white granite surfaces can be very hard on your eyes. The light bounces off them and can cause fatigue. A good pair of UV-blocking polarized lenses is best for eliminating the glare. If your glasses are loose fitting, consider a strap to secure them to your head. If you wear spectacles, clip-ons are good, but I prefer the convenience of the flip-up styles that I can work with one hand.

Hiking Poles   Hiking poles (also known as trekking poles) have been used widely in Europe for a long time and are now gaining popularity in the United States. Although a tree-branch walking staff à la Moses may be handy, who wants to carry an extra 4 pounds? Also, with a single staff, your body is torqued as you walk, which can stress your back muscles and lead to back issues. Poles work much better and help hikers of all ages improve power, endurance, and confidence on

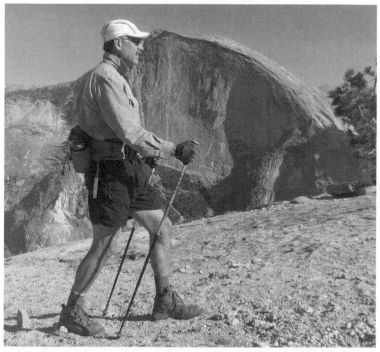

Hiking poles uphill

the trail. It's said that about 5% of the work of uphill hiking is transferred from the legs to the upper body when using poles. The poles will help you up the hundreds of granite steps, as well as provide stability when near cliffs. The best solution to the stress of hiking is the use of telescoping poles that adjust to your height. For optimum efficiency, the poles should be placed so that your elbows are at about hip level with about a 90-degree bend in the elbows. While traveling uphill, you can make the poles shorter and, conversely, while going down, you can extend them. Uphill, the poles are kept behind you to push off. Think of them as propelling you forward.

Poles are extremely helpful when going downhill. Remember that you may experience 5–6 hours of constant downhill hiking on the Half Dome hike. The poles should be extended and placed in front of you. This will absorb the shock and

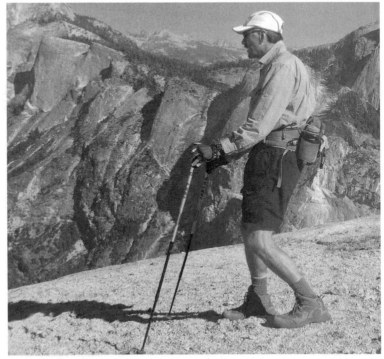

Hiking poles downhill

let your upper body do the slowing down instead of stressing your knees.

Hiking poles are better than ski poles because they're adjustable and much lighter. The poles have carbide steel tips, which grip the walking surface. Rubber tips are also available, but I do not recommend them on the granite trails at Yosemite. They tend to slip on the smooth rock.

Using poles can be a bit awkward at first. To help you understand the proper way to use them, I refer you to a great website focused on trekking-pole technique: **adventurebuddies.net.** The company produces two award-winning training DVDs (one for hikers and another for people with balance challenges) that will tell you everything you need to know about the use, care, benefits, and enjoyment you'll receive from using poles. Also, don't forget to bring Velcro straps to affix the poles (collapsed) to your pack when going up the cables.

Gloves I suggest using bicycle gloves with your trekking poles. Not only will these prevent possible irritation from your hiking poles, but the gloves will also protect your hands if you fall or decide to do some scrambling. When you arrive at the cables, I suggest switching to a pair of nitrile-dipped garden gloves. These tight-fitting gloves with breathable backs can be found at most hardware stores.

Raingear There is always a chance that it will rain during the months when the cables are up. While a good drenching may sound inviting when it's hot, if you get wet and chilled while hiking, your resistance may suffer and you may not feel at your peak. Be aware of hypothermia. If you take the Mist Trail next to Vernal Fall in early summer, you may get soaked within an hour of the start; in fact, you will get wet during the early season. How much depends on the amount of snow runoff. There are more than 700 steps on the lower Mist Trail, and the spray (or shower) off the fall can get heavy near the fall.

To stay dry, bring a cheap poncho from a surplus store—you don't want to carry a bulky jacket the entire day. You can stuff it into your pack and put it on before you enter the Mist Trail. I also suggest bringing two grocery produce bags and rubber bands to cover the tops of your boots so your socks don't get soaked. (I'll explain how to use them in Chapter 8 in the section on POI 2.) Often, I give my used rain outfits to others coming down the trail, so I don't have to carry them the rest of the day. Do *not* discard them on the trail. If you get no takers for your rain outfits, stuff them back into your pack. You might need them again if you encounter an afternoon rainstorm.

Cell Phones   Mobile phone coverage is hit or miss. The coverage and signal strength depend on your provider. The cell tower is behind the Valley Visitor Center, and in the shadow of Half Dome the signal is hidden. Most people are able to call home when they're sitting on top of Half Dome. You might want to make a quick call to say, "I made it!" A cell phone is a big asset in an emergency. Most rescues start with a call to 911. I advise turning off your cell until you need to make a call, as it may be trying to get a signal in the roam mode, which will drain your battery. As an aside, please don't bring two-way radios—reception is spotty, and they are noisy and quite annoying to hikers who are there for the serenity. Plus, why are you separated from your party anyway?

While we are discussing cell phones, I have made available a free smart device app that runs on iPhone, iPad, iPod Touch, and Android systems. It's a companion piece to this book and features how to prepare video segments on boots/foot care, water treatment, the use of hiking poles, and several other topics. I narrate the entire trail and tell historical vignettes.

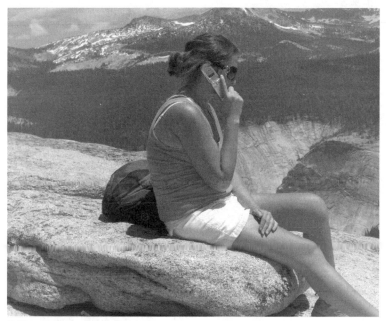

Calling Mom from the summit

One segment that you will certainly enjoy is the interview with Royal Robbins, the first person to climb the face of Half Dome in 1957. You can download the app through my website, **hikehalfdome.com**.

Flashlight/Headlamp   Carry a small (four AA battery) flashlight. June provides the maximum daylight, but hikers in September and October will find the sun setting much earlier. Remember that the sun will set even earlier than published because of the high mountains and heavy tree cover. The hike is no fun in the dark and is downright dangerous. Be prepared in case of an ankle sprain or other problems that cause delays.

Suntan Lotion   Apply a good coating of protection on your arms, neck, and face before beginning the hike. Bring a small sample-size tube for a midday reapplication.

Lip Balm   Your lips will welcome the relief in this dry altitude. Be sure to choose a balm with SPF protection.

Camera   The smaller, the better. Bulky cameras will get in your way, and you need both of your hands free. Having something around your neck will be a burden. Pocket-size digital cameras are ideal. Extra memory sticks and batteries will enhance your success.

Toilet Paper   Practice the old motto "be prepared." Camping stores carry small rolls that are not much bigger than a roll of quarters and will easily fit into your pack. The trail toilets at Yosemite are well stocked, but heed this advice for those unpredictable times.

Camping Gear   Toss in your sleeping bag in case the nights turn cold. Don't forget your earplugs, eyeshades, and balaclava (for head warmth).

Emergency Supplies

You'll be doing this particular hike on a well-marked trail, hopefully in less than 12 hours, but it is wise to be ready for the unexpected. The trails up to Half Dome are the most-used trails in the park, and help is usually readily available from fellow hikers or rangers walking the route, but don't rely on that. Be prepared to take care of yourself. If you do encounter trouble, don't have a cell phone, and cannot move, send word down with another hiker to dispatch help. A ranger station is located in Little Yosemite Valley, and rangers will have radios that can summon extra help if needed. Whenever I hike, I always carry a way for people to identify me in case I am injured.

You should bring along the following safety items:

First-aid Kit   Include moleskin or a similar protectant. Antiseptic, tape, Band-aids, aspirin, and so on should be included as well. Preconfigured hiking or biking first-aid kits are perfect. A small pocketknife will be handy. I prefer the type with tiny scissors and multiple tool attachments.

Identification Bracelet   One item that I wear all the time is a Medic Alert bracelet. I got it after a really bad ski accident resulted in major eye damage. I have my blood type and condition on it. Even if you have no medical issues, you should consider wearing one. Paramedics look for them. A simple ID bracelet is not a good idea—what if no one is home when they call? Medic Alert has a collect-call center to provide assistance. For a small annual fee, Medic Alert provides first responder access to my critical information worldwide (within privacy restrictions). It's nice to know that if I wipe out, I'm making it easier for medics to help me.

CHECKLIST

I suggest that you copy this list and go through it as you pack. Author's confession: On a trip years ago, my group got halfway to Yosemite and I realized I had forgotten to pack my boots! They were under the bumper of my car in my garage, and I didn't see them when I was packing. Home was a good 2 hours away, and traffic was getting worse with each passing mile. The night before leaving, I had mentally gone over what

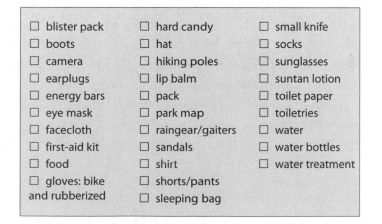

☐ blister pack	☐ hard candy	☐ small knife
☐ boots	☐ hat	☐ socks
☐ camera	☐ hiking poles	☐ sunglasses
☐ earplugs	☐ lip balm	☐ suntan lotion
☐ energy bars	☐ pack	☐ toilet paper
☐ eye mask	☐ park map	☐ toiletries
☐ facecloth	☐ raingear/gaiters	☐ water
☐ first-aid kit	☐ sandals	☐ water bottles
☐ food	☐ shirt	☐ water treatment
☐ gloves: bike and rubberized	☐ shorts/pants	
	☐ sleeping bag	

I needed to bring and must have skipped over the boots. We had to stop at an outdoor store for me to buy a new pair. Use the checklist!

When to Go

For hiking Half Dome, you can forget winter, early spring, and late fall. During those times it can snow in the valley, so just getting there could be a challenge. The major consideration is: "When will the cables be up on Half Dome?" They are usually up once the snows stop (May–early June), and they are taken down in the fall (October). The exact dates vary with the weather. I prefer to go in June because (1) after being inside during winter, it is a nice trip to look forward to; (2) the days are longest in June and allow plenty of daylight to complete the hike; (3) the waterfalls are full-flowing and spectacular; (4) there is less chance of a lightning storm early in the summer; and (5) the park is less crowded than later in the summer.

Guided Hikes

Some visitors prefer the security of doing the Half Dome hike with a skilled, permitted guide service. They know the trail, have first-aid training, bring water filters, and provide a fun experience. They will safely get you up the cables and will teach you a lot about the park. One-day and multiday hikes are offered. The services also go to other Yosemite destinations. Some of the local guide services include Lasting Adventures (**lastingadventures.com**), Southern Yosemite Mountain Guides (**symg.com**), Y Explore (**yexplore.com**), and the Yosemite Conservancy's Outdoor Adventures (**yosemite conservancy.org**).

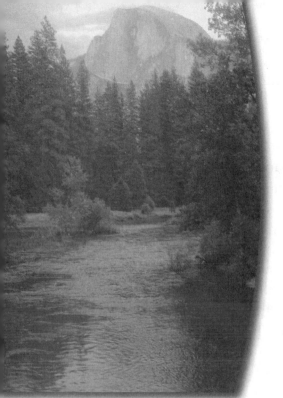

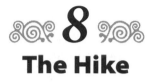 **8**

The Hike

Going to the woods is going home.

—**John Muir**

I use Curry Village as base camp for the hike because it is the most convenient sleeping and parking area. The often-published distance for the Half Dome hike is about 16 miles. Of course, the actual distance depends on where your starting point is and which route you take. The zero marker for my discussion is the logical start of the trail, next to the Merced River at Happy Isles. My cumulative distances and estimated hiking times are measured from there. I go from the trailhead to the Vernal Fall Bridge, up the Mist Trail, between Liberty Cap and Nevada Fall, through Little Yosemite Valley, up the John Muir Trail (JMT), then on the Half Dome trail and the cables. The return is via Nevada Fall and the JMT, skipping the Mist Trail. Total distance is 15.5 miles this way and not the 16 miles mentioned above. (This is explained a little later.) If you are staying anywhere other than in the general Curry Village area, you'll need to get to Curry Village and walk to the trailhead. You could take the Yosemite shuttle from any-where in the park and get off at stop number 16, Happy Isles. The big problem with this is that the shuttle buses don't start running until 7 a.m.

My pace is for a 10.5-hour round-trip, and this is the basis for the estimated times. Remember that time resting, enjoying the summit, and other diversions will affect your hike's actual duration. I've selected several points of interest (POIs), which are worthy stopping points and also will help you gauge how you're progressing. You may want to use a running chrono-graph as a general gauge for measuring how far it is between POIs. During the preparation of this guide, I used a state-of-the-art, hand-held Global Positioning System (GPS) receiver. This device allowed me to compile the trail measurements listed in the following sections. For your hike of Half Dome, I've done all the work; you do not need to bring a GPS. However, you may want to gain experience with your unit, and you can cross-check my readings. Altitudes may vary depending on just exactly where I hit the waypoint button. Also, I'm more than 6 feet tall; very accurate altitudes would be measured at ground level. The distances in this chapter were compiled off the GPS also. They are not as-the-crow-flies measurements but rather include actual distances cov-ered as I wound through the many switchbacks. The actual direct distance from Happy Isles to the top of Half Dome is less than 2 miles, but we will need to follow the trail on a counterclockwise route to reach our goal.

If you are traveling with four or more companions, it will be difficult for everyone to stay together. We all walk at different rates, anywhere from 2 to nearly 4 miles per hour, depending on the incline and on conditioning. Agree on a plan to meet up every hour or at the POIs described in this chapter. Make sure everyone has access to enough water, whether you carry it or

GPS PRIMER

In 1978 the United States initiated the Global Positioning System (GPS), primarily as a navigational aid to military operations. GPS is a network of 24 satellites orbiting the Earth at 6,000–12,000 miles out. In the 1980s the government made the system available for civilian use. Contact with at least three satellites is needed to calculate a two-dimensional position (latitude and longitude) and to track movement. With four or more satellites in view, a modern receiver can determine the user's three-dimensional position (latitude, longitude, and altitude) as well as track movement. From this, other information—such as speed, bearing, track, trip distance, distance to destination, sunrise/sunset times, and other data—can be calculated. Modern GPS units take advantage of hardware and software advances to yield accuracy within less than 20 feet even under dense foliage, in steep ravines, and in urban canyons. And now, many smart phones have GPS capability.

pump it. If you are taking small children, keep them close to you at all times. Have a plan for them if they do get separated from you. Tell them it's best if they stay where they are and ask other hikers for help. Giving them a whistle, just in case, is a good idea. Affix your name and contact information to them.

In the sections that follow, I'll describe the trail and POIs and give you the altitude, cumulative distance, elapsed time, and GPS coordinates for each. My times are only guidelines and may not apply to your hike. However, this information may be useful as another data point for you. I've included many photos, so you can see what a great hike you'll be enjoying, and the trail map on page 121 will give you a visual of your day.

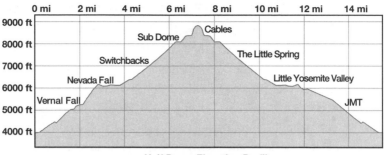

Half Dome Elevation Profile

Above is the hike's elevation profile. Use this when reading about the POIs.

Starting at Curry Village

Rise early and get organized—it helps to lay out your gear the night before. Use your checklist to make sure you don't forget anything. Have your breakfast and be on the trail by 6 a.m. A good goal is to arrive at the cables by 11 a.m. to avoid the crowds. An early start will allow you to make this an easy hike at your own pace, resting as you go along. Keep in mind this is a fun hike—not a death march! Remember, your pull up the cables will be much easier if you can zip right up, rather than inching up in traffic.

Hike east through the tent cabins until you reach the service road that the shuttle bus travels on. (Cars aren't allowed on this road.) You want to head toward Happy Isles, bus stop 16. As you approach the Merced River, look to the right, and you'll see the shuttle bus stop and a restroom facility. There will be many toilets farther on, so don't think this is your only chance to use the restroom. This is a good place to fill your water bottles.

Continue down the service road and turn right just after crossing the Happy Isles Bridge. The trail along the left side

Half Dome

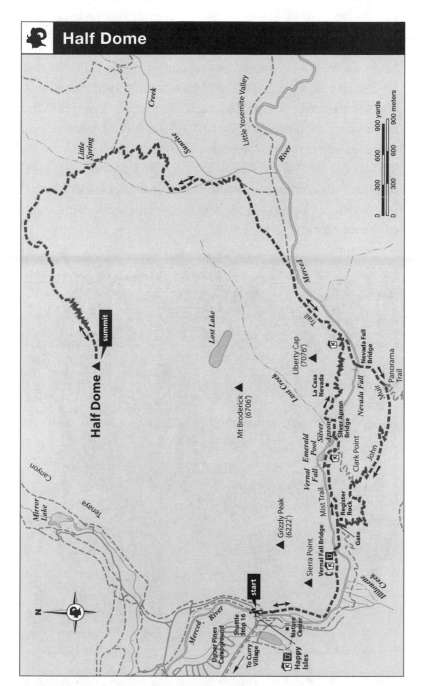

summit

Half Dome ▲

Little Spring

Creek

Sunrise

Little Yosemite Valley

River

Merced

Trail

Lost Lake

Liberty Cap
(7076')

La Casa
Nevada

Nevada Fall
Bridge

Panorama
Trail

Nevada Fall

Mt Broderick
(6706')

Lost Creek

Silver

Vernal Emerald
Fall Pool

Silver Apron
Bridge

Apron

Clark Point

John

Muir

Canyon

Mirror
Lake

Tenaya

Grizzly Peak
(6222')

Register
Rock

Sierra Point

Vernal Fall Bridge

Mist Trail

Gate

Illilouette Creek

start

Shuttle Stop 16

Upper Pines Campground

To Curry Village

Merced River

Nature Center

Happy Isles

N

0 300 600 900 yards

0 300 600 900 meters

of the Merced River will continue for about 200 yards, until you are just across from the Happy Isles area. On the river-bank, you will see a water-flow measuring station. This is the USGS river flow gauge station. Measurements are taken here and telemetered via satellite to USGS offices in Virginia. The roots of this station go back to 1915. In 1925 a continuous recorder was installed. Upgrades over the years have brought it to its current functionality and provide park officials with discreet and continuous water-quality data. The 1997 flood destroyed a bridge at the station, and you can see remnants of the foundation.

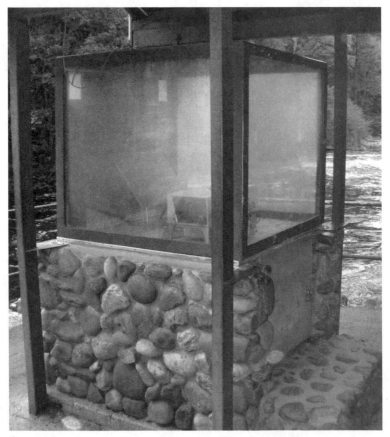

Gage station

Route Data

POI No.	Point of Interest	Elapsed time	Altitude feet above sea level	Odometer miles	Latitude North	Longitude West
1.	Mileage Marker Sign	0:00	4,093	0	37 43.859	119 33.500
2.	Vernal Fall Bridge	0:30	4,409	1.0	37 43.565	119 33.094
3.	Top of Vernal Fall	1:00	5,059	1.6	37 43.468	119 32.612
4.	Silver Apron Bridge	1:10	5,183	1.8	37 43.581	119 32.422
4a.	La Casa Nevada	1:40	5,313	1.9	37 43.624	119 32.284
5.	Mist Trail–JMT Junction	2:15	6,013	2.7	37 43.572	119 31.827
6a.	Little Yosemite Valley (enter)	2:20	6,146	3.2	37 43.753	119 31.639
6b.	Little Yosemite Valley (exit)	2:35	6,158	4.2	37 44.095	119 30.872
7.	Half Dome–JMT Split	2:50	7,005	5.1	37 44.705	119 30.771
8.	The Little Spring	3:15	7,231	5.9	37 44.878	119 30.879
9.	Base of Sub Dome	3:55	7,935	6.8	37 44.831	119 31.810
9a.	Top of Sub Dome	4:20	8,436	6.9	37 44.801	119 31.790
10.	Base of the Cables	4:30	8,395	7.1	37 44.777	119 31.855
11.	Apex of Half Dome	5:00	8,842	7.2	37 44.560	119 31.594
12.	The Little Spring —again	6:45	7,231	8.5	37 44.878	119 30.879
13.	Little Yosemite Valley —again	7:45	6,158	10.7	37 44.095	119 30.872
14.	Mist Trail–JMT Junction—again	8:15	6,013	11.7	37 43.572	119 31.827
15.	Nevada Fall Bridge	8:30	5,640	11.9	37 43.310	119 32.020
16.	Clark Point	9:00	5,548	13.2	37 43.502	119 32.696
17.	Vernal Fall Bridge —again	9:50	4,409	14.5	37 43.565	119 33.094
18.	Mileage Marker Sign —again	10:30	4,093	15.5	37 43.859	119 33.500

Note: Data will vary widely depending on your walking speed, how long you spend at each POI, how often you rest, time spent on the summit, accuracy of your GPS, and so on. Waypoints may differ from your readings, depending on where each is entered. Use this chart as a guide only. It may be copied for trail use.

GEORGE ANDERSON'S OTHER CONTRIBUTION
In the fall of 1881, George Anderson was given a $3,000 contract by the state of California to build a trail from the valley on the north side of the Merced starting near Happy Isles to the top of Vernal Fall. A motivation for Anderson may have been to create a trail to allow visitors to access his proposed hotel at the base of Half Dome. In 1882 he worked on the trail and got to just before the Vernal Fall Bridge. He invested much of his own money and intended to go up the left side of the Merced all the way to the top of Vernal Fall and opposite today's Mist Trail. Today the paved approach to Vernal Fall is his work. He died before it could be completed. As you approach the Vernal Fall Bridge, look to your left and up. You can see some of Anderson's work up the left side of the Mist Trail.

The expanse well behind this area was the site of the large rock fractures caused by rockslides, as discussed in the Introduction. You can view the talus field. Just to the left, you'll see the trail heading into the hills. You are now at the start of the famous JMT. Many people will be on the trail, so you won't get lost. Soon, you'll come upon your first photo opportunity: the mileage marker sign.

Mileage Marker Sign

POI
1

ELAPSED TIME . . . . 0 hours
ALTITUDE . . . . 4,093 feet
CUMULATIVE DISTANCE . . . . 0 miles
GPS COORDINATES . . . . . . .N 37 43.859 W 119 33.500

As you head up the trail, you'll very quickly see a large red-brown sign on your left, listing the mileage to many park destinations. This is the official start and end of your Half Dome hike. You will have to add all the walking you did from your bed to here for a complete mileage total. Turn on your GPS here. The Half Dome hike is listed as an 8.2-mile one-way journey. Thus, a round-trip would be 16.4 miles. However, taking that route, you would totally bypass the Mist Trail route and miss up-close views of the two high waterfalls. The most scenic hike, and the way I recommend, is via the Mist Trail when going up and on the JMT past Nevada Fall when returning, for 15.5 miles total. The return route is longer, but your knees will be spared the downhill steps of the Mist Trail. I strongly feel that the hike is actually easier going up since you are primarily using your leg muscles that have been conditioned for the hike. Downhill hiking places great strain on your knees. There's only so much you can do to strengthen the muscles supporting the knees. Hiking poles help in this regard, but I will trade the slightly longer route to skip the downhill Mist Trail and spare my knees. Even if your knees are not a problem, the Mist Trail is more hazardous negotiating the damp steps downward. The JMT affords you vistas of Liberty Cap, Half Dome, and Nevada Fall that you would miss if you took the Mist Trail both ways.

At the mileage sign, you'll also be able to see how far it is to other destinations, such as Tenaya Lake and Clouds Rest. Save these destinations for future hikes. Leaving the mileage sign, continue up the trail. Many people are going to Vernal Fall only, and you'll soon leave them behind. But expect to see dozens more crowding this part of the trail on your return at the end of the day, so take your photos now.

HIGH SIERRA LOOP TRAIL		
	MI	KM
VERNAL FALLS BRIDGE	0.8	1.3
TOP OF VERNAL FALL	1.5	2.4
EMERALD POOL	1.6	2.6
TOP OF NEVADA FALL	3.4	5.5
LITTLE YOSEMITE CAMPGROUND	4.3	6.9
GLACIER POINT	8.2	11.3
HALF DOME	8.2	11.3
CLOUDS REST	10.5	17.0
MERCED LAKE	13.1	21.0
TENAYA LAKE	16.4	26.0
TUOLUMNE MEADOWS	27.3	44.0
MOUNT WHITNEY VIA JOHN MUIR TRAIL	211.0	340.0
NO PETS ON TRAILS		

THE JOHN MUIR TRAIL

The John Muir Trail (JMT) was named for Muir after his death. He trekked along its path on his many journeys. The trail runs 211 miles on the crest of the Sierra Nevada mountains. Many people begin in Yosemite Valley and hike south to the top of Mount Whitney, the tallest peak in the lower 48 states at 14,495 feet above sea level.

The JMT is a must-do journey for avid hikers. After you've hiked Half Dome, you may consider tackling it someday. Plan on about 4 weeks to complete the trail. The JMT was the idea of Theodore Solomons, who suggested a trail along the spine of the Sierra. He hiked what would become today's trail with John Muir, Joseph LeConte, and other Sierra Club members. In 1914 the Sierra Club, together with the state of California, began trail planning, and after Muir died on Christmas Eve of that year, the trail took on his name as a way to honor him.

POI 2

Vernal Fall Bridge

ELAPSED TIME . . . . 30 minutes
ALTITUDE . . . . 4,409 feet
CUMULATIVE DISTANCE .1 mile
GPS COORDINATES . . . . . . .N 37 43.565 W 119 33.094

As you walk up the paved path you will get some good ups and downs to warm up. To your left you will a see large rockfall that at one time was the site of a trail to Sierra Point. It has long been closed and is not recommended for use. Rattlesnakes abound here, and it is pretty rough scrambling. Sierra Point was the one spot where you could see four waterfalls from a single vantage point: Vernal Fall, Nevada Fall, Yosemite Falls, and Illilouette Fall. Grizzly Peak lies just above you and to the left. You can easily see and hear the roaring Merced River to your right. As you continue, the view to the right will open up and you may catch a glimpse of Illilouette Fall streaming down in the distance. All the falls at Yosemite are fed by snowmelt and are virtually gone by late August, depending on the previous year's snowpack.

Once you arrive at the wooden footbridge, you can look up and to the left to see the waterfall framed by trees. An emergency telephone is nearby. A sink and water fountain provide the final opportunity to fill your bottles with potable water. For the rest of the hike, you'll need to treat the water.

Also, the restroom building at the right, opened in the 1930s, will provide your last chance to use a flushing, porcelain toilet. There are no trash cans, so please pack your waste.

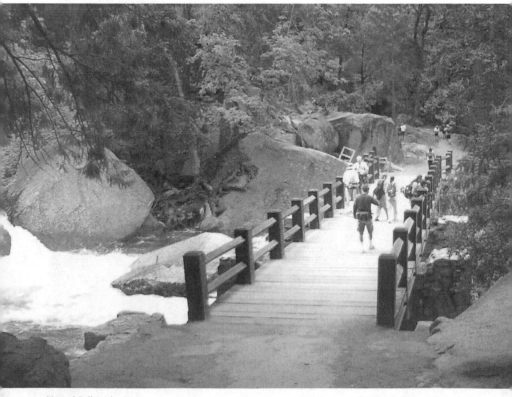

Vernal Fall Bridge

A couple hundred yards up the Mist Trail, you will arrive at a control gate. It is closed during the winter, when the steps ahead might be covered with ice. A junction here allows you to continue on the Mist Trail or go right onto the JMT. Regardless of which way you proceed at the control gate, look to your hard right, and just a few yards up the JMT you will see a large granite rock to the left of the trail. It is called Register Rock. In the early days before the government organized things, people built trails in the rough terrain and charged tolls to use them. For a period in the 1860s hikers signed or "registered" on the rock and paid a toll to use the trail to get to Glacier Point and Nevada Fall. The alternative was the Mist Trail, described below, but that involved navigating a scary series of ladders next to the fall.

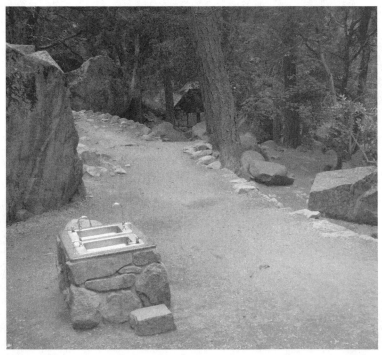

Last potable water

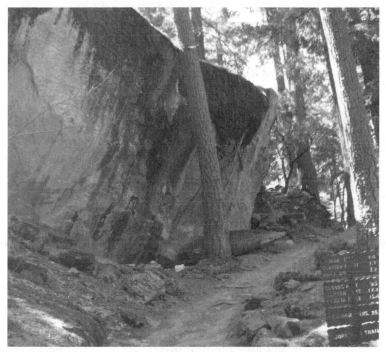

Register Rock

On a recent trip, I looked closely high on the rock and believe the following inscription could have been done more than 125 years ago: GERTRUDE SMITH 1881 F.K.C. It is too high to be modern graffiti, and it would have been very hard for a tagger to suspend himself by a rope and write it. I think Ms. Smith could have stood on the shack that once stood by the rock to write the inscription. Most of

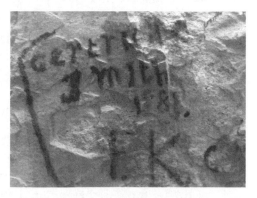

Possible historic inscription?

the historic signatures were lost when park superintendent Colonel Harry Benson ordered them removed in 1907.

I suggest you take the Mist Trail up during your morning hike. It will converge with the JMT at the Nevada Fall area. You will get wet from the spray on the Mist Trail in May and June, but it will be shorter than taking the JMT. The Mist Trail route to Nevada Fall is 2.6 miles versus 3.7 miles via the JMT. If you want to stay dry, the JMT is the way to go, but you will miss some interesting sights. Later in the day, we will return to Happy Isles on the longer JMT to save our knees from the downhill pounding.

Be forewarned: The lower Mist Trail will serve up nearly 700 steps, which will test how hard you trained. Your party will spread out into fast, average, and slow packs. Hiking poles will help you with the haul up.

Stop for 10 minutes every hour to rest and drink. When ascending the many steps, when you step up, lock your back leg briefly and put all your weight on it. As you step up, use momentum to swing the leg forward. Try to get a rhythm going as you walk. Counting cadence helps pass the time. "Left, left, left–right–left." Singing softly helps your breathing. Use your diaphragm to pump your air. If your knees ping, try going a little pigeon-toed. This moves the stress point and might help. Breathe through your mouth. You'll suck in more air. Exhale as though you are blowing out a birthday candle. This will allow you to breathe in more on your next inhale.

The Mist Trail in early summer can be a deluge, with the waterfall throwing off a shower onto the trail. It is very exciting and highly recommended. Watch for rainbows as the mist hits the sun. In May and June the spray will begin about halfway to the top. At that point, I put on my poncho (a cheap surplus store one) and gaiters made from produce bags. Simply go to your local supermarket and get the free plastic bags normally used for produce. Bring them with you on your hike, along with two rubber bands. Before you reach the spray, wrap the bags around the tops of your boots and secure them with the rubber bands. This will keep the water out of your boots. Another handy idea is to bring binder clips to secure your poncho to your hat brim and your pants. Without these, the wind will blow the poncho all around, and you may get soaked. If you wear your raingear, you'll be dry enough.

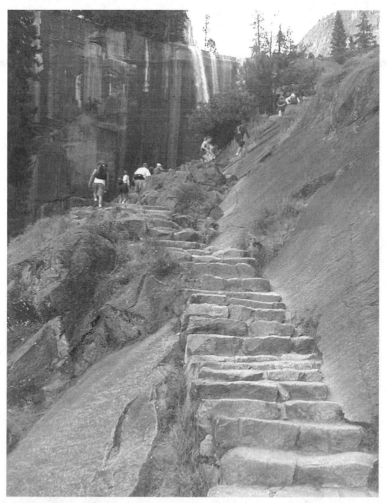

Mist Trail in September

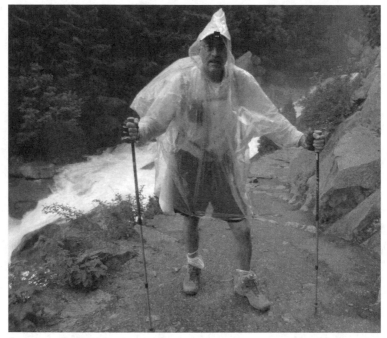

Gearing up for the deluge

Once you are through the spray, you can give your used raingear to others coming down the trail so you don't have to carry it the rest of the day. Do *not* discard it on the trail. If you get no takers for your raingear, stuff it back into your pack. You might need it again if you encounter an afternoon rainstorm.

Halfway up, an overhanging rock arch provides a brief shelter. Your trekking poles will steady your climb. As you head up the nearly 700 steps, pay homage to Stephen Cunningham, who constructed this difficult trail up to the cliff.

Near the top you will be out of the spray and can continue up the remaining steps. Off to your right you will see the Fern Grotto. This overhang is a quiet place to relax if you can negotiate the short climb up and have plenty of time. The huge gap was carved by dynamite, and visitors used wooden

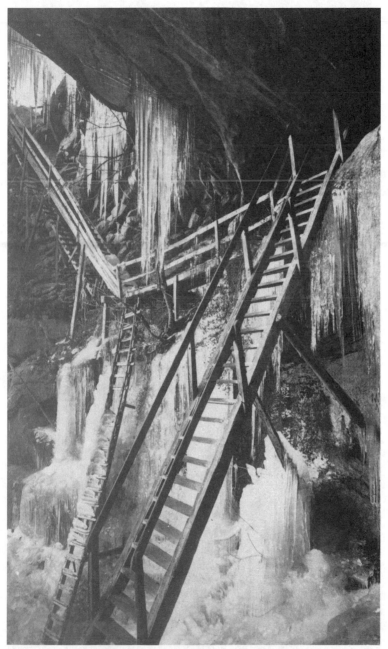

The original way to the top; courtesy of the Yosemite Research Library,
National Park Service

ladders to access it from 1858 to 1897, when stone steps were installed in place of the ladders. The original ladders, built by Cunningham, were in two sections: the first began beneath the overhang in Fern Grotto and led to a ledge midway up. From there, visitors took a short dogleg left to the second ladder, which led to the cliff top just south of Vernal Fall's summit. This two-part system was replaced in 1871, when Albert Snow erected a wooden stairway (with safety railings) to the top of the overhang. As you approach the very top, you'll ascend several steps carved into the rock. The handrails on the trail that exist through the exposed areas of the mist section of Vernal Fall were installed in 1929. They run alongside the river below the waterfall, along the cliff face, and at the apron atop the fall.

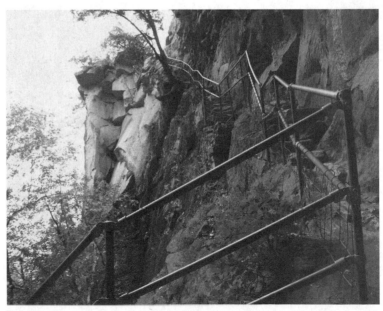

Today's railing system

Top of Vernal Fall

POI
3

ELAPSED TIME .... 1 hour
ALTITUDE................................... .5,059 feet
CUMULATIVE DISTANCE .... 1.6 miles
GPS COORDINATES .... N 37 43.468 W 119 32.612

Vernal Fall is a 317-foot-tall, 80-foot-wide symmetric fall that is postcard perfect. The viewing area here is superb. Fences will prevent you from accidentally going over, so you can safely snap several action shots. You can also glimpse your fellow hikers struggling up the Mist Trail. Take a rest here; you deserve it. Stay behind the rail and do not go near the water. In July 2005, a man climbed over the rail, stood in the water a mere 20 feet from the edge, and slipped over to his death. In 2011 Yosemite had a 200% snowpack, and the melt was long and strong. That July, despite warning signs and a protective fencing, ten people climbed over the rail, and three were swept over to their deaths.

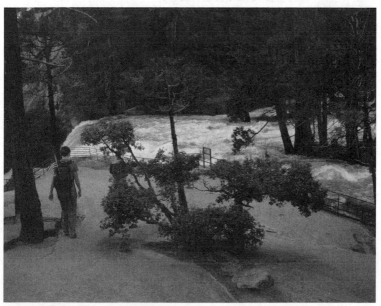

Stay behind the Vernal Fall safety fence.

After your short break, follow the trail signs and stay to the right of the river. You will soon see a composting outhouse uphill to your right. The toilets are well maintained and clean.

Through the trees to your left, you can see the Emerald Pool. It is a large bulge in the river with an inviting but deadly area that may seem like a fun place to swim. Swimming is prohibited due to the cold water, slick banks, current, and proximity to the fall just around the corner. Do not go into the Emerald Pool.

As you transition from a dirt trail and begin to hike up granite slabs, you will reach a confusing trail junction with two metal signs that both say NEVADA FALL. Go left; in fact, on the hike to Half Dome, when you arrive at a fork, always go left. Here, if you go right, you will get to Nevada Fall, but via Clark Point and the longer JMT. After passing the Emerald Pool, very shortly you will cross the wooden Silver Apron Bridge.

Silver Apron Bridge

POI	ELAPSED TIME . . . . .1 hour 10 minutes
4	ALTITUDE . . . . .5,183 feet
	CUMULATIVE DISTANCE . . . . .1.8 miles
	GPS COORDINATES . . . . .N 37 43.581 W 119 32.422

The Silver Apron Bridge is one of many that were built here over the years. The current bridge was rebuilt in 1997 after flood damage. It is 42 feet long and similar to the Vernal Fall and Nevada Fall bridges in design, with two 9-by-5-inch rails.

Remember the waterfall downstream? Under the Silver Apron Bridge, the Merced flows down a long, smooth, narrow chute and into the Emerald Pool. Although it is reminiscent of a waterslide, resist the temptation to go for a ride. The river tends to run fast through the narrow channel. Despite graphic warning signs, people sometimes unwisely go for a swim, which results in calls to Yosemite Search and Rescue.

Continuing on the trail, you'll soon be able to see Liberty Cap to your left (and up). Proceed toward Nevada Fall through a quiet forested area. As you bend to your right, keep your eyes out for a wide-open rocky space on mostly level ground on your right. Continuing, look for a rather open area just to the right of the trail. You'll see several large slickrock slabs. You have arrived at a fascinating place with an interesting history: the former site of La Casa Nevada hotel. Nothing remains of the hotel today except a few shards of glass. If you use your GPS at these coordinates (N 37 43.624 and W 119 32.284) at about 5,300 feet, you may see some of them. (For more on La Casa Nevada, see the sidebar on the next page.)

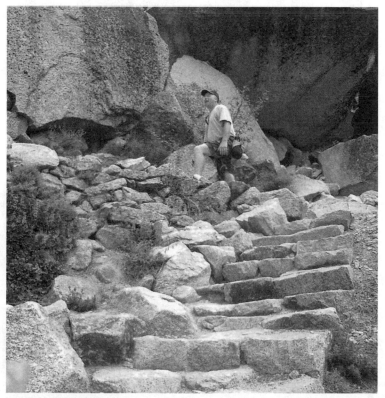

Upper Mist Trail steps

LA CASA NEVADA

In 1870 Albert Snow and his wife, Emily, operated a hotel that was originally called the Alpine House but later went by the name La Casa Nevada—a play on their name (in English it means The Snow's House). To allow access from the valley, in 1869–1870 Snow constructed a trail that switch-backed from Register Rock up to Clark Point and onto the flat area between Vernal and Nevada falls. The view of Nevada Fall from the hotel was recorded in photos and drew many visitors.

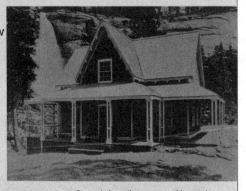

Snow's hotel; courtesy Yosemite Research Library, NPS

Some travelers stayed overnight before hiking to Glacier Point. Snow built two main buildings to accommodate guests. The first, built in 1870, was a one-story, rectangular building known as the Alpine House. By 1871 he had doubled its size, creating 12 rooms. By 1875 he had added the chalet, which had 10 bedrooms and a parlor, increasing his guest capacity to about 40. Snow even diverted the river to bring it closer to the property. Emily kept guests happy with her baked goods.

By 1889 the Snows began to feel the passage of time and became unable to maintain the hotel. Both died soon thereafter. The hotel operated under another owner until a fire destroyed it (like most other Yosemite hotels) in 1900. It was soon deemed a hazard, and all remnants were cleared out. In 1972 the Sierra Club cleared the site and placed historic artifacts in the Yosemite Museum.

As you approach the top of the trail, the view of Nevada Fall to your right is spectacular. You travel far enough away from the fall to stay dry but still get a pretty good up-close look at the 594-foot gusher. *Nevada* in Spanish means "snowy," and the white foam reminded early explorers of a cascade of snow.

As you proceed up, this area is reminiscent of the steep steps of the lower Mist Trail. Large granite switchbacks seem to go on forever. Gaze up at row after row of steps and appreciate the work it took to build these trails. You are now nestled between Liberty Cap and Nevada Fall. This leg is slowgoing, so rest occasionally and enjoy the view of Nevada Fall.

Mist Trail–JMT Junction

ELAPSED TIME .2 hours 15 minutes
ALTITUDE. . . . . .6,013 feet
CUMULATIVE DISTANCE . . . . .2.7 miles
GPS COORDINATES. . . . . N 37 43.572 W 119 31.827

Finally, you reach the top and rejoin the JMT coming from Nevada Fall. You're now starting to gain altitude. At this point, you are more than 2 miles from Yosemite Valley and less than 5 miles from Half Dome. The trail junction draws a healthy crowd of hikers in line at the two-unit composting toilet; the park does a great job of keeping the toilets on the trail clean and well stocked with toilet paper. Nevada Fall is just minutes to the right, but we will save it for our return at the end of the day. Take a short rest here; you are now approaching the halfway point of your hike to the top. When you're ready, continue to the left and head toward Little Yosemite Valley.

Little Yosemite Valley

POI
6

ELAPSED TIME .2 hours 20 minutes
ALTITUDE. . . . . .6,146 feet
CUMULATIVE DISTANCE . . . . .3.2 miles
GPS COORDINATES. . . . . N 37 43.753 W 119 31.639

The trail now eases to a gentle walk in the park. You soon enter a lightly wooded area on a clearly marked trail. Don't wander off the trail because this will accelerate erosion. Occasionally look up to your left; you'll see your goal: Half Dome.

Little Yosemite Valley was once a thriving summer village for the Native Americans in the area. Named by the first whites to see it, this valley extends toward Merced Lake. The 2,000-foot-high walls sculpted by glaciers resemble the majesty of the main Yosemite Valley.

You will be on the level trail for only about a mile, so enjoy a brief rest after the steep climb up the Mist Trail. The Merced River slowly meanders to the right of the trail. It is a good,

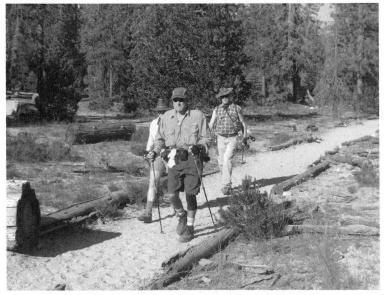

Little Yosemite Valley

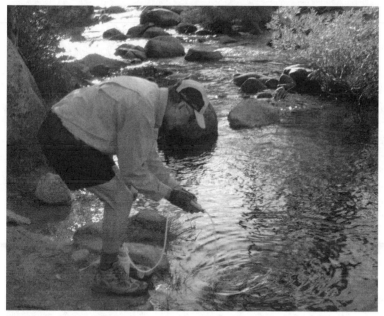

Filtering at the Merced

safe place to filter water. You'll have only one more chance before Half Dome, so drink what you have and replenish both bottles. Don't be tempted to drink directly from the clear, babbling brook. Remember the giardia discussion? I begin adding electrolytes at this water stop. Also, be wary of the Steller's jay, an aggressive species of bird that lives in this part of the park and will take a sandwich right out of your hand.

The fall is far downstream, so the water is calm. You could go for a swim if you were not on a mission to Half Dome. A quick look up and to the left reveals the back side of Half Dome. You can clearly see the main hump and Sub Dome. The cables are hidden from this vantage point. Continue down the sandy trail and pass the sign for the backpacker lot.

This campsite is for backpackers with wilderness permits. Some hikers elect to stay here and do the Half Dome summit in two days. While this would afford an early trip to the top, permits are limited and competitive. Additionally, campers must carry their gear up the 2,000 feet from the valley. This area is known for its bear activity, but don't worry; no one has ever been killed by a bear at Yosemite. A large (and the last) four-unit composting outhouse is located to the right.

Farther down is a ranger station that supports this area of the park. On another day you may want to continue up the river toward Merced Lake and the High Sierra Camp there. A lottery is held each year for overnight slots at the five High Sierra Camps. Spaced about 8 miles apart, they are a rewarding day hike and welcome you with tent cabins and hearty meals.

Once past the backpacker camp, you'll reach the forest and begin the slow steady grind uphill. You will know you are still on the correct route when you see a sign reminding you that you cannot camp above 7,900 feet. Got that permit?

The trail soon begins a series of gentle switchbacks, taking you in and out of trees. You'll be taking your sunglasses on and off, but generally this is not a sunny hike. Just get in a groove with your hiking poles and enjoy nature at its best. Smell the Jeffrey pines, the white firs, and cedars.

Half Dome–JMT Split

ELAPSED TIME	2 hours 50 minutes
ALTITUDE	7,005 feet
CUMULATIVE DISTANCE	5.1 miles
GPS COORDINATES	N 37 44.705 W 119 30.771

When you are ascending this forested area, you may be lucky enough to see mule deer—easily recognized by the shape of their ears, which actually do resemble mules' ears. They like the heavy brush and tree cover here and frequent the main valley meadows. More injuries have been inflicted on park visitors by mule deer than by black bears. A fully grown buck can weigh up to 400 pounds. Don't feed them! With so many deer in this stretch, you can rest assured that mountain lions are on the lookout for a meal. To give you peace of mind, no one has been killed by a mountain lion in the entire state of California since 2004, and it's estimated that only 5,000 of these animals are left in the state. They are also called pumas, cougars, or panthers and can range upward of 250 pounds. It is extremely rare to see one, so if you do, cherish the moment. Hunting of anything in a national park is prohibited

Rattlesnakes are also common here. If you stay on the main trail, you will be fine. Be cautious if you take a potty break (100 feet minimum from a trail or water). There are 14 types of snakes in the park, but only the western rattler is venomous. They have a flat triangular head and are colored cream to black with splotches. Bites are very rare, but if you hear a rattle, move!

The endless series of switchbacks continue upward at a steady pace. Don't veer off the main trail. Be alert; it will be easy to mistakenly take the trail to Clouds Rest. The trail compass bearing is 330 degrees, so you're almost due north and circling around the back of Half Dome. Watch for the metal trail sign pointing the way to Half Dome in 2 miles. The main trail splits to the right and continues as the JMT toward Clouds Rest. You should head left on the Half Dome trail.

The Little Spring

ELAPSED TIME . . . . 3 hours 15 minutes
ALTITUDE . . . . 7,231 feet
CUMULATIVE DISTANCE . . . . 5.9 miles
GPS COORDINATES . . . . N 37 44.878 W 119 30.879

The switchbacks will seem to go on forever, so rest often and drink before you are thirsty. Nibble as you go. Pay close attention to this POI. It will help you find a little-known water source. Some guidebooks refer to a stream that lies off to the right a couple hundred yards. Don't bother trying to find it. You will soon walk within mere feet of a reliable spring. It doesn't have an official name, so I call it the Little Spring. It is always flowing, albeit only a few inches deep and not bigger than a tabletop, but since it is not snowmelt, you can count on it to be running. You must be alert to locate the Little Spring on your left. After you make a hard left switchback turn, watch for a downed tree that lies with its roots facing the trail. I've walked by it when talking or daydreaming. Study the photos of this area.

Water that runs through soil and sand is usually safe to drink, but I still recommend you use a water purification system before drinking from this spring. Remember the deer mentioned earlier? Other animals use this water source and can

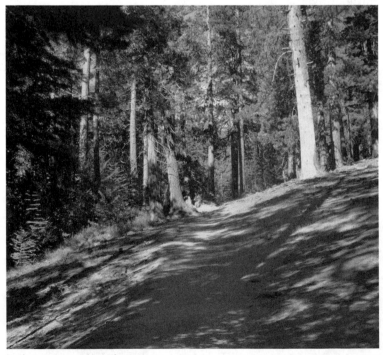

Trail view approaching the spring

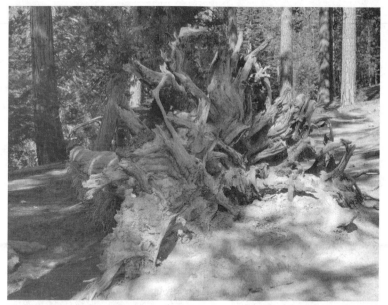

Look for these roots to help you find the Little Spring.

contaminate it. Giardia and *Cryptosporidium* are linked to E. coli in feces. These intestinal parasites must be treated or you will get very sick and could even die.

I have gotten water at the Little Spring the entire summer hiking season—as late as October. The spring is small and shallow, so do not stir up sediment. Hold the filter inlet just below the surface to avoid getting sediment into your filter and clogging it. Filling up here should allow you to get to the top of Half Dome and back to this spring before you need to refill. Drink heartily here, adding electrolytes, and then refill your bottles before continuing. Don't underestimate the difficulty that lies ahead. Use the GPS coordinates if you can't find the spring.

Here's a Mr. Half Dome tip: Since this is the last water source between here and the top, I bring an empty 2-quart bladder— not a hydration pack, but a flexible container that I can stuff into my pack. I then fill it, attach a nylon strap to it, and carry it over my shoulders for the next hour. When I am near Sub

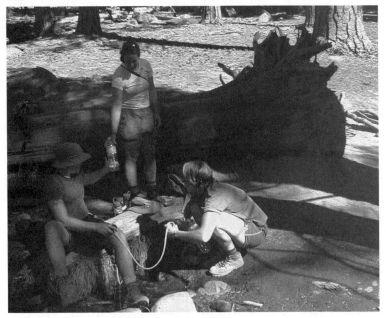

The last water between here and the top!

Dome, I hide it in the woods; then after I return down the cables later, I can retrieve it and enjoy those 2 quarts to get me back to the Little Spring.

Base of Sub Dome

POI
9

ELAPSED TIME .3 hours 55 minutes
ALTITUDE. . . . . .7,935 feet
CUMULATIVE DISTANCE. . . . . .6.8 miles
GPS COORDINATES. . . . . . . .N 37 44.831 W 119 31.810

You continue on a series of switchbacks in the shade of the forest. About 0.5 mile beyond the Little Spring, you will get a glimpse of Sub Dome with the back side of Half Dome looming above it. The trees get thinner, and the views open up. When you emerge from the trees, you will finally see the profile of the back side of Half Dome in full.

You have now gained enough altitude to see many of the surrounding formations. You will know you are near the base of

Sub Dome when a large flat area appears and several downed trees provide "benches" to enjoy this nice resting place. Many people kick back and regroup in the shade. Since there are no more toilets, you should make a final stop in the woods before proceeding. Remember to go at least 100 feet from the trail. Dig a 6-inch-deep cathole if needed and pack out your toilet paper. *Note:* There are no toilets or places to go up top.

As you proceed up toward the base of Sub Dome, a ranger may be present to check your permit. He or she can ask for your permit even if you are coming down. If you didn't come up the face, you need a permit. If you have one, you may proceed up the long grind of Sub Dome.

Although this formation is not specifically named on maps, the rangers indeed call it Sub Dome. Incorrect names include Quarter Dome (a formation near Clouds Rest), the Granite Staircase, the Switchbacks, and even the Shoulder. The most understated part of the entire hike is the 400-foot rise up Sub

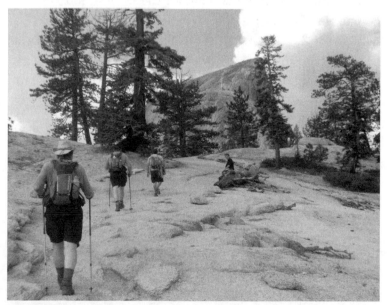

Half Dome is in sight.

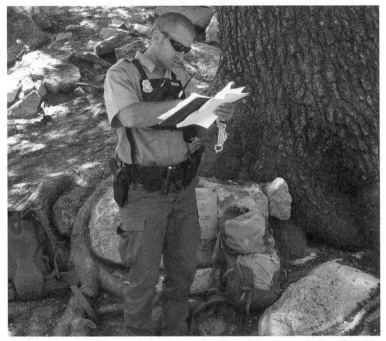

Ranger checking permits

Dome. Many say it is harder than the cables. Sub Dome is composed of a bidirectional switchback granite staircase that was carved in 1919 when the cables were erected and was improved most recently in 2005. It lies above the tree line and is very strenuous. It can take 45–60 minutes to get to the top of Sub Dome.

Most steps are narrow and require single-file passage. This stretch consists of more than 800 granite steps of varying sizes. Some are just a few inches tall, while others are nearly a foot high. The actual total vertical rise is about the same as the trek up the cables. The trail twists precariously, so care must be taken. This imposing area is actually part of the bigger Half Dome rock, but because it is much smaller, it is often not given as much respect. Move over and let the downhill hikers by; they have momentum and you deserve a rest. Hiking poles help with the push up and provide stability on these tricky steps. The steps die out about three-quarters of the way up, and you must watch for people descending to ensure you don't lose your way. If no one is approaching, simply aim for the highest part of the rock. A slow and steady pace is best. Pause often to enjoy the view. You'll be very tired when you reach the top of Sub Dome.

Once at the top of Sub Dome, you can gaze down into the saddle of Half Dome and then up to get a good view of the famous cables. If you've kept pace, it should be about 11 a.m., and you'll be rewarded with finding a reasonable number of other hikers on the cables. If you have arrived after noon, you'll probably see some congestion. Before the permit process, I saw people waiting for 45 or more minutes just to get on the cables.

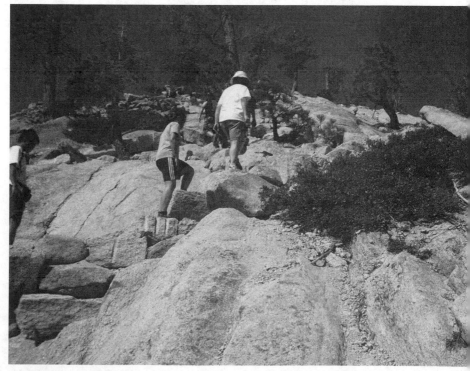

The Sub Dome knee grinder

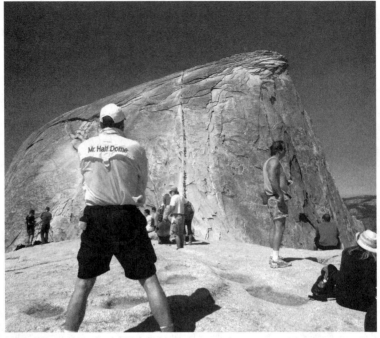

Mr. Half Dome here (in spirit) to help you.

Base of the Cables

POI	ELAPSED TIME . . . . 4 hours 30 minutes
10	ALTITUDE . . . . 8,395 feet
	CUMULATIVE DISTANCE . . . . 7.1 miles
	GPS COORDINATES . . . . N 37 44.777 W 119 31.855

When you finally arrive at the top of Sub Dome, you'll come face-to-face with the infamous cables. Photos do little to convey the task that lies ahead. Assuming you are doing well, sit back, rest, tighten your laces, drink, and secure your poles, bottles, and camera. The depression just before the cables is called the saddle. Here you get an appreciation of the steep areas to the left and right (I call them Infinity and Oblivion). At the base of the cables, you may find several pairs of old gloves discarded by those who went before you. They are trash, pure and simple; they are not put there as a public

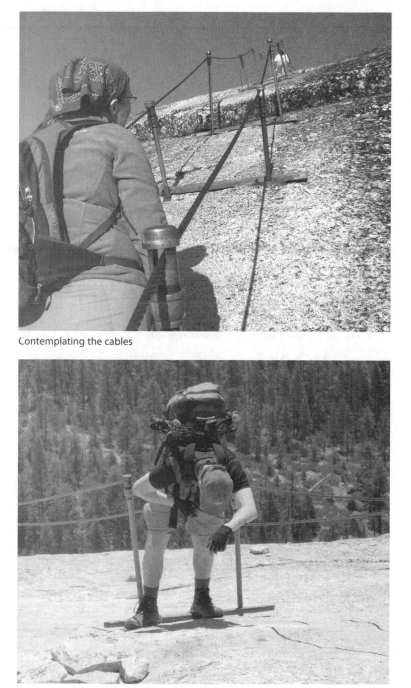

Contemplating the cables

Rest as needed.

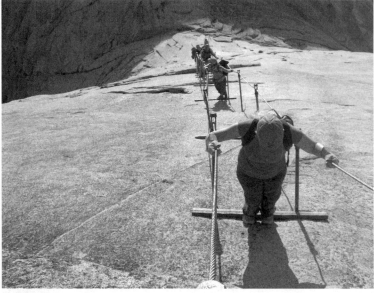

Don't look down!

service. The park service discourages this type of littering; in fact, they'd appreciate you taking a few pairs with you.

Here, I change out of my bicycle gloves and put on my rubber-coated ones. Collapse your poles and attach them securely to your pack. If you have faith in your fellow humans, you may try leaving your gear near a rock, but beware, the squirrels will gnaw at your pack to get to a snack.

You should estimate your total trip time and turn around if you are beyond your halfway time. From here it can take a long time to get up and back down the cables, depending on the crowd. You do not want to risk night hiking.

First, a word of caution: If there is any storm activity nearby, or you get the smell of rain, DO NOT go up. Lightning can travel up to 10 miles from its cloud source, and those steel cables conduct electricity. In 1985 two men died after a lightning strike up top. Besides lightning, rain makes the granite very slippery, and the wind can numb your hands, creating deadly consequences when attempting to descend. In 2011 a woman was killed when she was apparently shocked while descending the conductive steel cables, lost her grip, and slid down the damp rock.

You'll notice that there is no ranger or authority to control who goes up. No age limits, no weight limits; just free passage to anyone willing—true American freedom. When you have your courage up, go for it! The cables are multistranded steel, about 5/8-inch in diameter, and have more than enough strength. They are attached to 3-foot stanchions (support poles) and resemble a banister. The poles rest in holes drilled into the rock. Note that I said "rest." They will come out if you pull up on them. After this happens to you the first time, you'll forever treat them gingerly. At the base of every pole pair is a long 2-by-4-inch piece of wood placed perpendicular to the path. This allows you to stand every 10 feet and take a rest.

From the base to the top is a 425-foot vertical rise. The safest strategy here is to keep three points in contact at all times (hands and feet alternating between cables and rock). You'll get a better grip from your boots if you maintain a flat foot against the rock, rather than walking on your toes. Your leg muscles are large, and you'll fare better if they do most of the work. The use of a homemade harness with clips is not recommended. If you fall, you may slide down 10 feet to the next pole while hitting your head and garroting your body. A nylon strap has little give, and the sudden stop could hurt your back. If you intend to use a harness, get a real mountain-climbing one that goes around your waist and thighs. You also need two shock-corded straps with two carabiners. The rig is called a via ferrata. You will need to release and reclip 68 times going up and coming down. You should practice this a lot before your trip. It will take a very long time.

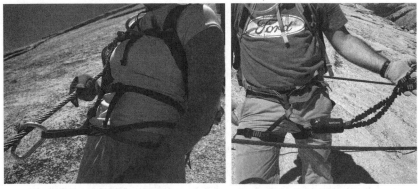

Bad: Home-made harness   Good: A via ferrata

I do not recommend pulling out a camera for panorama shots while ascending. If you must take a picture, have the camera around your neck to minimize this insecure interval. If you are scared (who's not?), try not to look out. Focus on the 10 feet in front of you. Breathe deliberately, but don't hyperventilate. This is a difficult climb, but you can do it. About halfway up

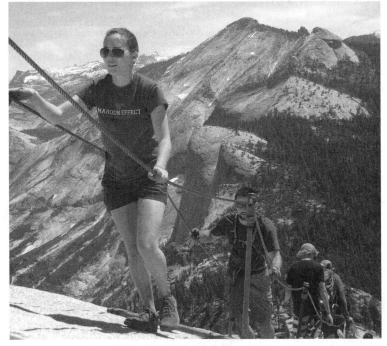

Upward! Clouds Rest in the background

the rock, you'll encounter discontinuities in its surface; this means you'll have to be prepared to step over these granite ledges. Be aware, also, that a couple of times, the cable that you are clutching will descend back to the rock and end to be replaced by a new run of cable. (Each side of the cable system is actually several connected runs of cable anchored to the rock, not one continuous piece.) The transition of the cable as it drops down the rock can give you pause.

The cable route is bidirectional. You'll have to lean out of the way so those coming down can pass. Be cautious of other hikers with large backpacks. They may be unaware that their pack is swinging wide as they pass you. You don't need an unexpected bump to throw off your concentration.

Climbing Technique

Many people use both cables to pull up. While this technique is fine in the beginning, I find that it primarily uses the pectoral muscles. I prefer to use a single cable and rappel up. Crouch and keep your feet flat to maximize friction.

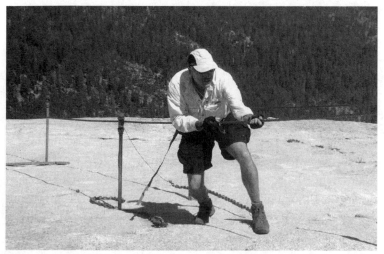

Try the rappel technique.

It will be hard to use your legs at the 45-degree angle, so pull yourself up using your back, shoulder, and core muscles. Go from board to board and rest. Pin your foot against the pole to brace yourself until the next board is available. Try not to get stuck between boards, as this will make for a harder climb. Don't gaze out if you are afraid of heights. There is no one in charge, and there are no rules. In America we stay to the right side ascending and descending. Be polite but keep moving. People may suffer anxiety attacks; it's ok to politely pass them.

Eventually, you'll see the rock slowly end its steep slope, and you'll be able to walk unaided but breathless. Depending on the traffic, this may have taken you 15–45 minutes. Congratulations. You did it!

Bonus: On my free Half Dome smart device app (see **hike halfdome.com**), I include the footage of my ascent wearing a head-mounted camera. (It's also on YouTube. Search for "Half Dome Cables All the Way Up.") You can see the entire ascent in less than 12 minutes in living color!

Apex of Half Dome

```
ELAPSED TIME ............................... 5 hours
ALTITUDE.................................8,842 feet
CUMULATIVE DISTANCE......................7.2 miles
GPS COORDINATES........N 37 44.560  W 119 31.594
```

Work your way to the very apex of the rock. Bask in your accomplishment; high-five your mates. Enjoy your lunch and take a nap in the hot sun. Use your cell phone (it should work) to call your friends back home. Cautiously explore the rock and gaze down on the valley. The views are spectacular: the Yosemite Valley, Glacier Point, El Capitan, Clouds Rest, Tenaya Canyon, the Quarter Domes, Mount Watkins, Mount Hoffmann, and others. Bring your park map to help locate these sights. Be cautious of loose gravel on the surface. Be very aware of the edge and don't approach it too closely. Half Dome is surprisingly large: the surface approximates 17 football fields.

The far western end reveals a series of cairns or trail ducks (human-made rock stacks) and little else. There are few trees left on top of Half Dome; most were cut for firewood decades ago, when camping was allowed.

Find a quiet spot away from the crowds and imagine what it was like on top for George Anderson or John Muir. When you are ready to explore, the curved western dome reveals wildflowers and rock formations.

On the northeastern side, be careful near the face. Wall climbers may be coming up, so please don't toss anything over the side. Near the apex is the Visor, a popular photo

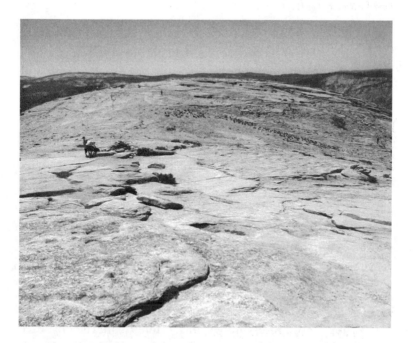

It's surprisingly big up top.

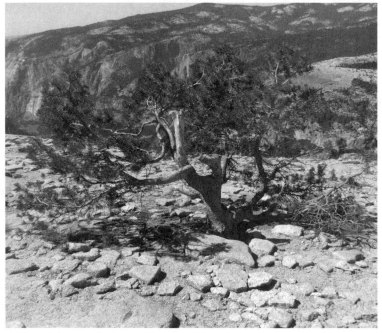

One remaining tree shrub

spot. This is often erroneously called the Diving Board. Although there are a few rocks that jut out, the true Diving Board is on the lower northwestern side of Half Dome and is where Ansel Adams took his famous black-and-white photos of the rock.

You'll see many interesting things up top. On one trip I was able to film a man proposing to his fiancée on the Visor. Watch for marmots and squirrels—they can actually climb up Half Dome! (The yellow-bellied marmot can grow up to 5 pounds.) Please do not feed these cute critters. They need to forage for themselves, lest they starve once all the tourists leave in the fall.

Let's discuss the great view from nearly a mile above the valley.

The Valley   Yosemite Valley spans 7 miles from the entrance near Bridalveil Fall. It's about a mile wide. From this vantage, it is easy to see how the three major glacier periods created the

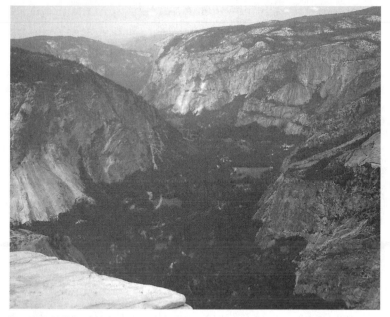

Yosemite Valley

shapes we see today. It was from near Bridalveil Fall (hidden around to the left) that the Mariposa Battalion first laid eyes on Yosemite in 1851. As you look to the west you can make out the haze of the great San Joaquin Valley, breadbasket to much of the country. The Merced River eventually merges with the San Joaquin, and its waters feed the farms. The first whites tried to keep many of the Native American names for the majestic sights, but the words were just too hard for the Anglos to master, so the names we have today stuck. The rock you are standing on now was called Tissiack by the Native Americans. Legend tells us that a Native American woman named Tissiack was walking in the valley near Mirror Lake with her husband, Tokoyee. They argued and began fighting. She threw her basket of acorns at him. The spirits were displeased, and he was turned into North Dome. The basket became Basket Dome, and Tissiack was turned into Half Dome. You can see a cameo of a woman on the face of the rock with tears running down her face.

El Capitan   It is fittingly named to represent the power of the rock itself and was known to the Native Americans as Tote-ack-ah-noo-lah. Their legend has it that one day two bear cubs were playing in the area and a huge rock began to rise up to the sky. Soon the bears were alone at the top of the 3,000-foot wall. The other animals could not get up to them until an inchworm slowly made its way to the top. He was too late, and the bears starved, but he brought back a rib bone to prove he made it. Today El Capitan is a mecca for big-wall climbers who climb the face, taking several days. It was first scaled in 1958 by Warren Harding, Wayne Merry, and George Whitmore in 47 days. Today's speed climbers are able to get to the top in less than 3 hours. In June 2010, Alex Honnold climbed Half Dome and then El Cap in 8 hours!

Glacier Point   Rising 3,000 feet above the valley, Glacier Point is accessible by foot via the Four Mile Trail and the Panorama Trail or by vehicle off CA 41. It provides the best all-encompassing views of Yosemite Valley, Tenaya Canyon, Half Dome, and Vernal and Nevada falls. It was the site of the famous Firefall, a summer spectacle that was held from 1872 until 1968. Each evening at 9 p.m. in season, burning embers were pushed over the edge of Glacier Point to the cheers of visitors. (For more information on the Firefall, see the sidebar on page 86.)

The Ahwahnee   The Ahwahnee Hotel is at the east end of the valley and is a five-star lodge. It was named in honor of the Native Americans that the Mariposa Battalion first met. They were the Ahwahneechee, which loosely means "those who lived in the place of the gaping mouth" (the valley). The hotel was the brainchild of the first NPS director, Stephen Mather. He knew that for the park to succeed financially, it would need a luxury hotel in keeping with the grandeur of

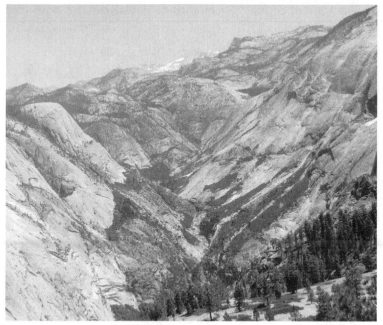

Tenaya Canyon

Yosemite. The hotel was opened to the public in 1927 at a cost of $1.5 million.

Tenaya Canyon   At your feet is the rugged Tenaya Canyon. Running to the northeast, it is a hazardous place with smooth granite walls carved by glacial action. Hiking the canyon is dangerous and not advised. Far to the north is Tenaya Lake, named in honor of the old chief of the Ahwahneechee.

Clouds Rest   The sharp peak to the right of Tenaya Canyon is Clouds Rest. The hike to the top takes about 7 hours round-trip if you start at the Tenaya Lake trailhead. It is much longer from Happy Isles. There are plenty of water sources en route. The hike up the spine is harrowing because it is only several feet wide. Upon arriving at the top of the nearly 10,000-foot peak, one can gaze down at the cable route of Half Dome. Just to the north and below lie two granite bumps called the Quarter Domes.

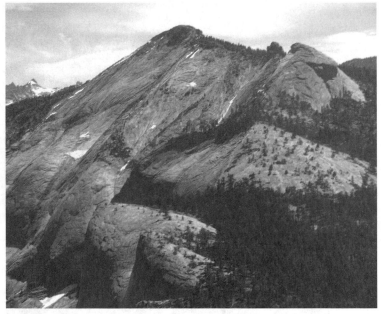

Clouds Rest

Mount Dana Far out to the horizon lies Mount Dana, the second-highest peak in Yosemite at more than 13,000 feet (Mount Lyell is higher). Mount Dana is named after James Dana, a 19th-century geologist who made important contributions to the geologic understanding of the Sierra Nevada. It is also known for having a small receding glacier at its summit, as does Mount Lyell. You can hike up Mount Dana by parking at the Tioga Pass park entrance and following a crude trail to the top.

Merced Canyon Looking back toward the cables you can see the vast Merced Canyon. The Merced River is fed from rain and melting snows in the higher elevations that flow to Merced Lake. A High Sierra Camp is located next to the lake.

Descending the Cables

After about 45 minutes on top of Half Dome, you will be ready to hike back. Many people descend facing downhill. I

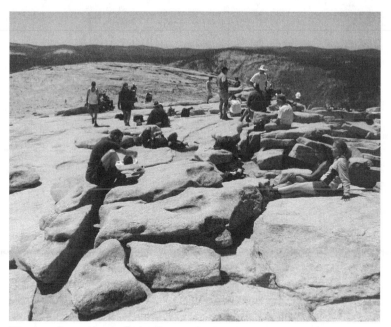

Friends gather on the top for lunch.

do not recommend this, as you will have to look at the scary rock below you, and your body's center of gravity will be rocking you forward. Also, all your body weight will be on your wrists. Good old gravity helps make going down the cables easier than going up. I suggest facing the rock as soon as it starts to get steep. A good way to go down the cables is to face slightly uphill and rappel down, just as you went up. The people coming up will gladly lean over so you can get by; they are pretty tired. If you feel any vertigo or a panic attack coming on, stop and breathe slowly. Inform your companions and slowly descend. You may try sitting down and sliding while holding on to the cables.

Next comes Sub Dome. Be careful of your footing and use your hiking poles to descend like a mountain goat. Always maintain three points of contact. The gravel surface can cause you to slip if you aren't careful.

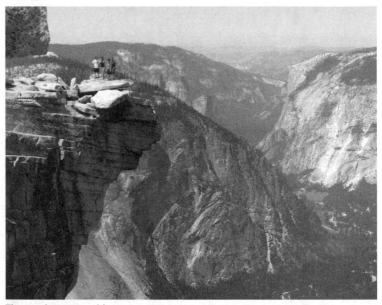

The overhang resembles a visor.

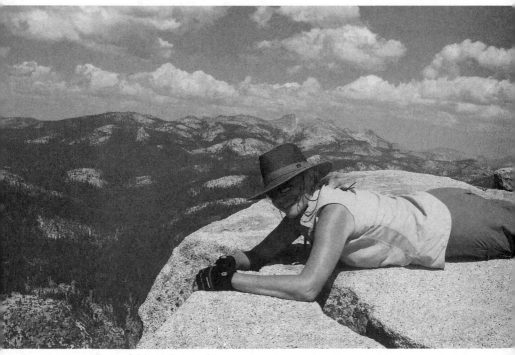

Be careful, but take a peek.

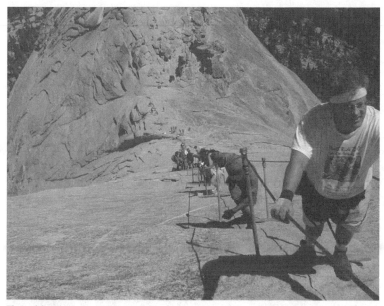

The cables down await you.

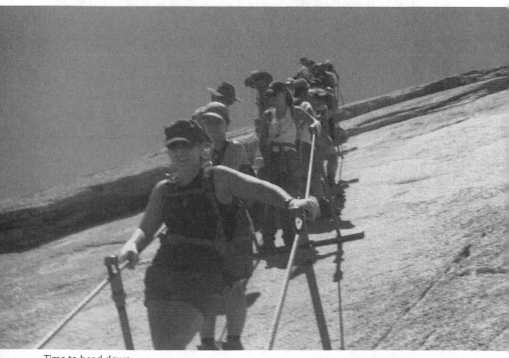

Time to head down.

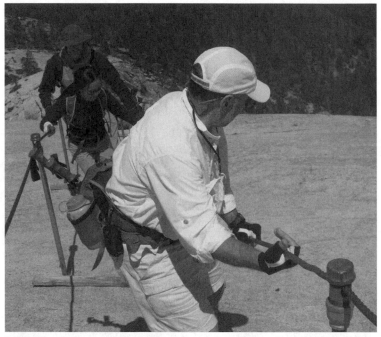

Try the "face up" rappel.

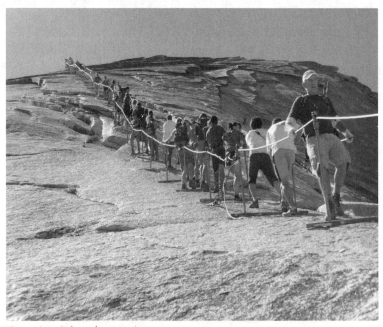

The rock is slick—take your time.

The Little Spring—again

ELAPSED TIME . . . . .6 hours 45 minutes
ALTITUDE. . . . . .7,231 feet
CUMULATIVE DISTANCE. .8.5 miles
GPS COORDINATES. . . . . . . .N 37 44.878 W 119 30.879

Less than an hour after leaving the dome, you'll once again see the Little Spring—now on the right side of the trail. You'll probably be carrying two drained water bottles by now. Fill them here, have a big drink, take a short rest, and keep going. You'll be seeing the same scenery on the way down that you saw on the way up, so I won't cover it again. This will be true until you take the JMT instead of the Mist Trail back. Your knees will thank you. A comment about the trip down: It can be harder than the trip up. The stress on your knees will take its toll. Also, don't underestimate the length of the return. After a couple of hours, you'll think Curry Village is just around the next switchback—not so! Pace yourself and resist the temptation to run down (you'll see a few doing so).

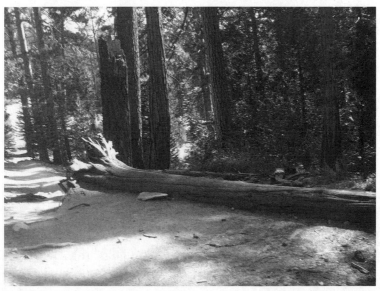

The Little spring as viewed going down.

Running downhill is really, *really* bad for your knees. Keep drinking and moving.

Little Yosemite Valley—again

ELAPSED TIME . . . . .7 hours 45 minutes
ALTITUDE. . . . . .6,158 feet
CUMULATIVE DISTANCE. . . . . 10.7 miles
GPS COORDINATES. . . . . N 37 44.095 W 119 30.872

Don't be tempted to run or crosscut trails. Crosscutting destroys the natural ability of the trail to hold water during rain and will cause it to erode faster. After you complete the last of the switchbacks, you come out of the woods and settle into Little Yosemite Valley. The trail forks; go to the right. This is the most direct path. If nature calls, take the left fork, and you'll soon see the large, elevated wooden facility. You may see a trail sign pointing to the backpackers camp, which also leads to the toilets. This "mother of all johns" has four units available. These toilets don't get as much action as the others on the trail, so the odds are high that you'll find no lines. Ok, back on the trail. Catch another glimpse of the Merced to your left and continue.

Mist Trail–JMT Junction—again

ELAPSED TIME . . . . .8 hours 15 minutes
ALTITUDE. . . . . .6,013 feet
CUMULATIVE DISTANCE. . . . . 11.7 miles
GPS COORDINATES. . . . . N 37 43.572 W 119 31.827

You're back now to the intersection of the two routes down: the Mist Trail or the JMT. You'll see many people converged here. Decision time: The longer (maybe a half hour more) route via the JMT or the shorter but steeper route via the Mist Trail? Unless you have a time-critical reason for going the Mist Trail, don't. Your knees will explode! There's really nothing to prove now. You already conquered Half Dome! Take the left trail; the sign at this point indicates 3.7 miles on the JMT to the valley. Head to Nevada Fall, just a few minutes' walk away. Look to your right and see Liberty Cap, then look down, and you'll see the trail leading to Vernal Fall.

Nevada Fall Bridge

POI
15

ELAPSED TIME .... 8 hours 30 minutes
ALTITUDE .... 5,640 feet
CUMULATIVE DISTANCE .... 11.9 miles
GPS COORDINATES .... N 37 43.310 W 119 32.020

Nevada Fall Bridge has undergone numerous reconstructions, most recently in 1997, because its location bears the brunt of severe storms. Its original log design was replaced in 1962 with a steel Bailey bridge that lasted 35 years before being lost to a storm in 1997. The current bridge features

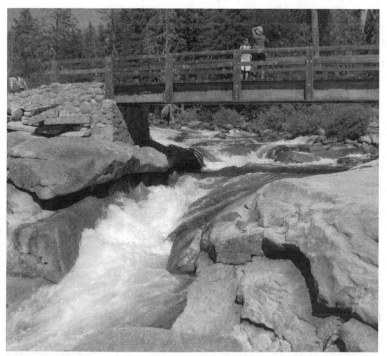

Nevada Fall Bridge

steel stringers and is modular enough that sections, such as rails and decks, can be replaced individually.

This is a good spot to kick back and recharge. The waters above the fall are usually packed with Half Dome veterans and others who did the day hike up from the valley. Take your shoes off and soak a bit. *Caution:* Do not go out into the placid-looking waters. There are deep holes and strong currents away from the shore. The rocks are slippery, and you can see what lies 50 yards downstream—Nevada Fall. It stands at 594 feet, and occasionally, somebody accidentally goes over. Treat some water and fill your bottles if needed and have an energy bar. Before crossing the bridge, go down to the right side (it's fenced) to an overlook and gaze at the power of the water going over the edge. Continue across the bridge and stay on the JMT. The Panorama Trail will join from the left.

A few yards down the JMT and you will be on the Rock Cut. The cliff area with water seeping out of it has been called both the Rock Cut and the Ice Wall. It was created to shorten the hike up to Glacier Point. The sharp drop to your right provides an unobstructed view of Nevada Fall, Liberty Cap, and Half Dome.

When the trail was built in 1931, dynamite was used to blast the path out of the rock. It was difficult to find men with experience or the intestinal fortitude to hang off the slope to set up dynamite plugs. Establishing the Rock Cut involved dynamiting a trail-width bench along 750 feet of granite. This construction was considered the most difficult and dangerous ever accomplished in trail work in Yosemite National Park. The project was orchestrated by the park's trail master, Gabriel Sovulewski. From 1908 to 1936, Sovulewski's achievements in the park's mountain trail system were culminated in the Rock Cut.

ASPHALT ON THE TRAILS

As you hike, you may notice what looks like old asphalt paving on the trails. Beginning in the 1920s, stretches of trails were sprayed with oil, or asphalt emulsion, in an attempt to limit erosion and provide a less dusty walking surface. While technically it's not hot-mix asphalt, the surface has hardened to an asphaltlike consistency.

Unfortunately, over time the surface has broken down, leaving large potholes and abrupt drop-offs, and rather than controlling erosion, the hardened surface has furthered it by not allowing natural percolation of water through the soil. In many places, the trail was refreshed annually with an application of oil to reduce dust. The trail's bituminous surfaces have not been maintained and have been eroding severely, creating tripping hazards, runoff channels, and puddling, as well as detracting from the historic character of the trail and being visually intrusive in a forest environment. I was quite surprised to see a fresh coat of oil put on the Happy Isles to Vernal Fall trail in the mid-2000s.

In decades past, people would use ice axes to climb the ice flow during winter; however, this is no longer permitted. Hike along the cliff and look back at Nevada Fall for a superb view. To the left of Nevada Fall is Liberty Cap. It has gone through several names, including Sugar Loaf Dome, Gwin's Peak, Mount Frances, Bellow's Butte, Mount Broderick, and others. Its current name comes from its resemblance to the knitted caps worn as far back as the Roman Empire. The caps were worn by commoners and stood for liberty. In 1865, while on a visit to Yosemite, California Governor Leland Stanford (yes, *that* Stanford) gave it the name The Cap of Liberty when he saw the resemblance to Miss Liberty on an 1871 silver dollar.

Between Nevada Fall and Liberty Cap is the upper Mist Trail—that rubble field is what you went up in the morning! It was originally a zigzag horse trail that suffered constant rockfalls and was almost abandoned. Behind Liberty Cap is a small valley containing Lost Lake, a large marshy area. This is the way to the Diving Board and a wall climb called Snake Dike—it's for experienced climbers only. The region between Lost Lake and the Diving Board becomes very rugged, with talus, cliffs, gullies, and dense forests of manzanita.

Look farther left and you will see Mount Broderick and then the back side of Half Dome. You can make out Sub Dome and the saddle, but the cables are just out of view. Grizzly Peak is the last formation as you pan toward the valley. Continue down the switchbacks—29 of them to the bottom.

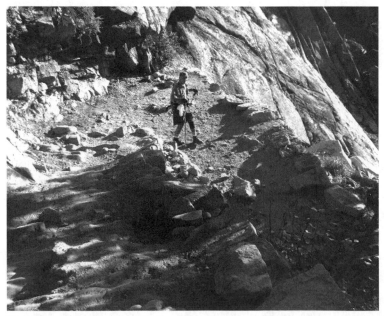
29 switchbacks ahead

Clark Point

ELAPSED TIME . . . . 9 hours
ALTITUDE . . . . .5,548 feet
CUMULATIVE DISTANCE . . . . 13.2 miles
GPS COORDINATES . . . . N 37 43.502 W 119 32.696

You'll approach a trail split at Clark Point—watch for the interpretive sign. This overlook affords a good view of Nevada Fall and the canyon across the river. If you were to take the trail to the right, you would end up back near the Emerald Pool— too long for a quick return to your base camp. It does feature an unusual view of Vernal Fall to your left, but save this for another hike. The run of switchbacks down from Clark Point historically had the name Porcupine Switchbacks. This long, winding series of switchbacks was originally repaired

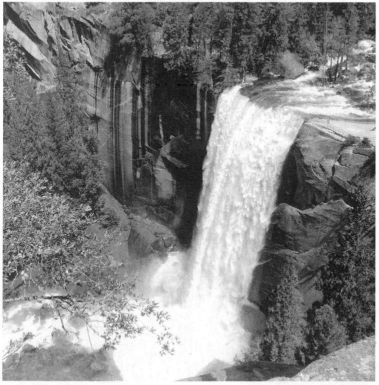

Vernal Fall viewed from below Clark Point   © Scott Gehrman

GALEN CLARK

Clark Point was named for Galen Clark, "guardian of Yosemite," who was appointed by the commissioners for day-to-day administration of the park. When he was 39, Clark caught tuberculosis and moved to the Sierra forest near Wawona to live out his remaining projected six months. But he recovered and stayed, later stumbling upon the Mariposa Grove of Big Trees. He spent years teaching others to respect nature and worked with Senator John Conness to develop the legislation that became the Yosemite Grant that President Lincoln signed in 1864. Clark served in the capacity of guardian of the park for 24 years in the time before the formal National Park Service was formed. He later wrote three books about Yosemite and died in 1910 at the age of 95. Mount Clark and the Clark Range are also named after him.

in 1931, and many rock retaining walls were added. A large rockslide in 1986 damaged some sections of these walls, but all were rebuilt.

After reading the signage at Clark Point, go left and continue down an uneventful trail that is occasionally traveled by

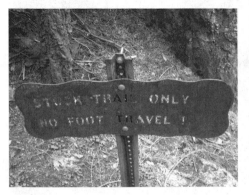

sure-footed pack animals. Give them the right-of-way. These very intelligent mules and horses can find their way back home by leaving little trail markers behind them; watch your step. Soon you will hear the rushing Merced River. You

Keep right!

will eventually reach a metal sign that instructs foot traffic to take a right fork. Left is for pack animals, and that route would add a lot of distance before you got back to Happy Isles.

Next you will pass Register Rock and rejoin the lower Mist Trail. The footbridge will be crowded, and you are very close to the end of your trip.

Vernal Fall Bridge—again

ELAPSED TIME . . . . .9 hours 50 minutes
ALTITUDE . . . . .4,409 feet
CUMULATIVE DISTANCE . . . . 14.5 miles
GPS COORDINATES . . . . N 37 43.565 W 119 33.094

Bring it home now. You've merged with the Mist Trail and are back to the bridge. The flush toilets will be on your left, and the water fountain will be on your right. Get one last water refill. This area will be mobbed in the late afternoon, and you'll be glad you got all your pictures this morning.

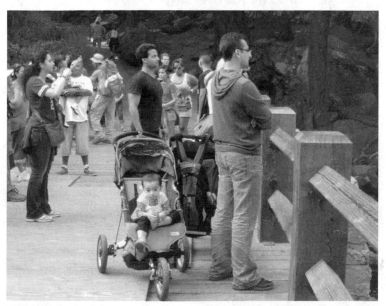

Yes, even baby strollers!

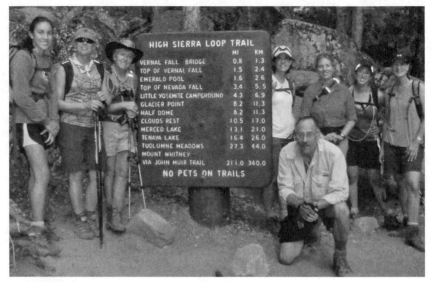

High Sierra Loop Trail sign:

HIGH SIERRA LOOP TRAIL	MI	KM
VERNAL FALL BRIDGE	0.8	1.3
TOP OF VERNAL FALL	1.5	2.4
EMERALD POOL	1.6	2.6
TOP OF NEVADA FALL	3.4	5.5
LITTLE YOSEMITE CAMPGROUND	4.3	6.9
GLACIER POINT	8.2	11.3
HALF DOME	8.2	11.3
CLOUDS REST	10.5	17.0
MERCED LAKE	13.1	21.0
TENAYA LAKE	16.4	26.0
TUOLUMNE MEADOWS	27.3	44.0
MOUNT WHITNEY		
VIA JOHN MUIR TRAIL	211.0	340.0

NO PETS ON TRAILS

End of a long day

POI
18

Mileage Marker Sign—again

ELAPSED TIME .... 10 hours 30 minutes
ALTITUDE.....................................4,093 feet
CUMULATIVE DISTANCE.................... 15.5 miles
GPS COORDINATES........N 37 43.859 W 119 33.500

After running the gauntlet of casual hikers, you reach the unofficial end of the adventure—the mileage marker sign and Happy Isles. Congratulations! You have officially completed the Half Dome hike in one day. You can now head back to your tent or hotel room. I suggest you do some slow stretching of your quads, calves, and hamstrings. Then get to the shower and directly to dinner. You will sleep well and possibly suffer leg cramping, depending on how much preparation you did. Sore muscles are caused by lactic acid and will go away. Gentle walking helps move the acid around. Tomorrow you can get your "I made it to the top" T-shirt. Now plan your next adventure. Carpe diem!

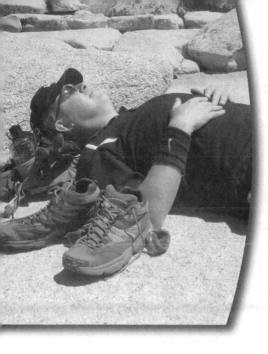

9
Epilogue

Keep close to Nature's heart... and break clear away, once in a while, and climb a mountain or spend a week in the woods. Wash your spirit clean.

—**John Muir**

Post Hike

You'll be tired after hiking Half Dome. After a quick celebration, I suggest you head to the showers. They are located near the main complex of Curry Village; showers and towels are free for guests. Hot water is plentiful, but the sheer mass of humanity and the trail dust carried in can make the showers messy.

After your shower, walk over to the Curry Pavilion buffet or the Pizza Patio. If you want to see a different part of the valley, take the shuttle bus to the main Yosemite Village. You can dine at Degnan's Loft or the Deli, or venture over to the Yosemite Lodge and enjoy its Mountain Room Restaurant. Dinner at the Ahwahnee is a real treat. Built in 1927, this National Historic Landmark features historic architecture on a grand scale. Be aware that the evening dress code here calls for no jeans or shorts. Most park eateries close at 9 p.m., so plan accordingly.

I hope you enjoyed this book and that it helps make your journey a bit easier. Keep in mind the myth about Milo picking up that calf every day! Make Half Dome an annual hike—the place is fantastic. And check my website for updates to the book: **hikehalfdome.com.**

See you on top! Carpe Diem!
Rick Deutsch "Mr. Half Dome"

Appendix 1

Key Dates in Yosemite and Half Dome History

1833	Joseph Walker's party views valley from Yosemite Point.
1851	Mariposa Battalion enters Yosemite Valley.
1853	Article in *San Francisco Herald* extols virtues of Yosemite Valley.
1855	James Hutchings leads tourist party into Yosemite Valley.
1855	Thomas Ayres publishes lithographs of the region.
1856	The Coulterville Trail establishes a western access along Bull Creek and Tamarack Flat to the valley.
1857	Galen Clark discovers Mariposa Grove.
1857	Stephen Cunningham builds the first ladders up Vernal Fall at Fern Grotto.
1858	Stephen Cunningham builds trail from valley to top of Vernal Fall, using the old Indian trail on the south side of the Merced.
1859	First photographs taken of Yosemite Valley by Charles Weed.
1859	James Hutchings and Charles Weed attempt to climb Half Dome.
1861	Carleton E. Watkins photographs sites in Yosemite.
1863	California Geological Survey begins survey of Yosemite area.
1864	Yosemite Grant: Congress deeds 48 square miles of Yosemite Valley and Mariposa Grove of Big Trees to State of California.
1864	Eight commissioners, led by Frederick Law Olmsted, appointed to oversee Yosemite Valley and the Big Trees.
1867	Bridge built across river above Vernal Fall, enabling easy access to top of Nevada Fall.
1866	Galen Clark is Yosemite's first guardian; remains until 1879.
1868	John Muir first visits Yosemite.
1869	Guardian Galen Clark grants Stephen Cunningham permission to build toll trail from Register Rock to flat between Vernal and Nevada falls.
1869	Opening of the Transcontinental Railroad improves access to Yosemite.
1870	Albert Snow's hotel (La Casa Nevada) built above Vernal Fall, with a view of Nevada Fall.
1870	Diamond Cascade Bridge built near site of today's Silver Apron Bridge.
1871	John Conway builds trail from La Casa Nevada to top of Nevada Fall and attempts to climb Half Dome.

Key Dates in Yosemite and Half Dome History

1871   Stephen Cunningham erects ladders next to Vernal Fall; Albert Snow later adds wooden staircase.

1872   Firefall off Glacier Point begins.

1874   Coulterville (June 17) and Big Oak Flat Road (July 17) completed into the valley from west and north, respectively.

1875   Wawona Road (CA 41) completed into the valley from the south.

1875   October 10, first ascent of Half Dome by George Anderson.

1875   Sally Dutcher (first woman), Galen Clark, and John Muir climb Half Dome.

1877   Selah Walker reportedly took the first photograph on the top of Half Dome: a fuzzy shot of George Anderson.

1879   George Wheeler party surveys and maps Yosemite Valley.

1882   State purchases Vernal Fall stairway for $300 from Albert Snow.

1882   The state (Yosemite Valley Commission) buys Mist Trail for $300.

1882   George Anderson builds trail from Happy Isles to bridge below Vernal Fall.

1884   George Anderson dies; buried in Yosemite Cemetery.

1884   Alden Sampson and A. Phimister Proctor restring rope on Half Dome.

1889   Snows cease operating La Casa Nevada due to ill health. D.F. Baxter operates it for 2 years; then it closes for good.

1890   Yosemite National Park created. CA retains valley and Big Trees.

1891   U.S. Army (Buffalo Soldiers) administers Yosemite.

1892   Wooden staircase and railings replace ladders next to Vernal Fall.

1892   Sierra Club organized by John Muir.

1898   Camp Curry opened by David and Jenny Curry.

1900   Fire destroys La Casa Nevada; park later clears debris.

1900   First automobile enters Yosemite Valley.

1903   President Theodore Roosevelt meets John Muir at Yosemite.

1905   California redeeds Yosemite Grant to United States.

1907   Yosemite Railroad makes first scheduled run.

1908   Rockslide destroys most of the Nevada Fall Trail.

1913   Damming of Hetch Hetchy signed into law by Woodrow Wilson.

1913   Automobiles permitted into park.

1914   Department of Interior civilian employees replace Army administration.

Key Dates in Yosemite and Half Dome History

1914	John Muir dies in Los Angeles of pneumonia.
1915	Stephen T. Mather oversees all national parks.
1915	Appropriation made for John Muir Trail.
1915	Tioga Wagon Road bought from the Bennettville mining company.
1916	National Park Service Act approved.
1917	National Park Service organized as bureau of the Department of the Interior.
1919	A.C. Pillsbury takes first aerial photos of Yosemite.
1919	M. Hall McAllister funds construction of Half Dome cables system on behalf of Sierra Club.
1923	Hetch Hetchy Reservoir completed.
1926	All-Year Highway (CA 140) from Merced to Yosemite opens.
1927	Ahwahnee Hotel opens.
1928	Asphaltic products used on the Vernal-Nevada falls trails.
1931	Rock Cut Trail built from Nevada Fall toward Clark Point.
1932	Wawona area added to the park (14 square miles).
1933	Wawona tunnel opened.
1934	Comfort station built at Vernal Fall Bridge.
1934	Civilian Conservation Corps replaces cables on Half Dome.
1935	New Glacier Point Road completed.
1940	Current Big Oak Flat Road opened with three tunnels into valley area.
1945	Yosemite Railroad assets sold for scrap; all tracks removed.
1956	Liberty Cap Gully switchbacks rebuilt after winter flood destruction.
1956	New Yosemite Lodge completed.
1957	Fish hatchery building at Happy Isles converted to nature center.
1957	First climb of face of Half Dome led by Royal Robbins.
1958	First climb of face of El Capitan led by Warren Harding.
1964	Congress passes the Wilderness Act, ensuring areas of solitude devoid of human impact.
1967	Liz Robbins becomes the first woman to climb the face of Half Dome.

Key Dates in Yosemite and Half Dome History

1968	Firefall off Glacier Point abolished.
1969	McCauley House and Glacier Point Hotel burned.
1980	Yosemite General Management Plan released.
1984	Yosemite named World Heritage Site; 94% of park designated as wilderness.
1990	Mr. Half Dome, Rick Deutsch, completes first hike to Half Dome summit.
1997	100-year flood brings 8 feet of water to valley; major trail, bridge, and area damage.
2000	First snowboard descent of Half Dome's east side by Jim Zellers.
2005	Major work done on the trail up Sub Dome.
2007	*One Best Hike: Yosemite's Half Dome* makes its publishing debut as Half Dome's first comprehensive guidebook.
2008	More than 1,200 people go up Half Dome cables on weekends.
2008	Alex Honnold free-solos the Regular Northwest Face of Half Dome in 2 hours and 50 minutes.
2008	Ryan Ghelfi runs the entire Half Dome hike, round-trip, in 2:30:50.
2009	Half Dome Cables Modeling and Visitor Use Estimation Final Report
2009	Half Dome Stewardship Plan announced for 2-year development.
2010	Permits required to go up Sub Dome and the Half Dome cables on Friday, Saturday, Sunday, and holidays.
2010	Rickey Gates runs the entire Half Dome hike, round-trip, in 2:28:18.
2011	Permits required every day for going up Sub Dome and the Half Dome cables.
2012	Permits via lottery initiated for going up Sub Dome and Half Dome.
2012	Long-Term Half Dome Stewardship Plan review continues.

Sources
Arthur C. Pillsbury Foundation: acpillsburyfoundation.org
A Century at Yosemite (1851–1960), Cantor Arts Center and Stanford University Libraries.
Gerdes, Marti M. Nevada Fall Corridor: A cultural landscape report. Master's thesis, University of Oregon, 2004.

Appendix 2

Preventive Search and Rescue Tips

Yosemite Search and Rescue (YOSAR) is the primary group tasked with aiding lost and injured visitors. YOSAR responds to approximately 250 incidents in the park each year; nearly one-third of those incidents happen on trails leading to Half Dome. Preventive Search and Rescue (PSAR) provides services and guidance to help visitors avoid problems. Below is PSAR's advice to Half Dome hikers.

Know your fitness level. The hike from the trailhead at Happy Isles to the summit of Half Dome gains 4,800 feet in elevation and is 14–16 miles, round-trip, depending on which route you choose (the Mist Trail is 1 mile shorter, but much steeper, than the John Muir Trail). It takes an average of 10–12 hours to hike to the summit and back. Honestly assess the fitness level of each member of your group. High altitude and hot summer temperatures may exacerbate preexisting medical conditions; be well rested and well hydrated, and eat plenty the day before the hike.

Plan to start your hike before sunrise and have a non-negotiable turnaround time. For instance, if you haven't reached the top of Half Dome by 3:30 p.m., you will turn around. Check for sunrise and sunset times before you hike. Each person should carry a flashlight or headlamp with fresh batteries.

Be prepared for cool temperatures and rain. The summit is typically 15°F–20°F (8°C–11°C) cooler than Yosemite Valley, and windy conditions are common. Bring raingear and extra clothing layers. If you become soaked, head back to the trailhead instead of trying to wait out the storm—the only way to stay warm is to keep moving.

Do not continue up Sub Dome or Half Dome if storm clouds are overhead, if you hear thunder or see lightning, if it is precipitating, or if the ground is wet. If you are on the summit with a storm moving in, leave the area immediately (while still using caution when descending the cables and steps). Please see the next page for additional information on what to do in the event of a storm.

Drink plenty of water. Suggested minimum amount is 1 gallon (4 liters) per person. The only treated water on the trail is available at a drinking fountain at the Vernal Fall Bridge (less than a mile from the trailhead). Merced River water is available up to Little Yosemite

Valley; we recommend you treat any water collected from a natural source before drinking it. Choose slow-flowing, non-slippery access sites when collecting water from the river; a good spot to get water from the river is just before reaching Little Yosemite Valley, where the trail closely parallels a relatively calm section of the river.

Eat snacks regularly. Salty foods help replace the salt lost through sweat. Make sure everyone in your group has food and water with them in case you get separated.

Pay attention to how you're feeling. If you're huffing and puffing, you are working harder than you should. Take water and snack breaks in the shade.

Designate meeting areas for your group. Identifying meeting areas can help reunite the group if members become separated while hiking.

Stay on the trail. Do not take shortcuts off the trail or across switchbacks. Besides causing trail erosion and being illegal, cutting switchbacks is a major safety hazard. Bring a good topographic map and compass and know how to use them.

Most accidents and injuries happen to hikers on their way back to the trailhead. Pace yourself and continue to take breaks. Pay attention to the trail; hikers generally lose the trail on their way back down, hardly ever on their way up.

KEY POINTS RELATED TO STORMS AND LIGHTNING

- The Half Dome Trail is not closed during bad weather or during predicted bad weather. Hikers are responsible for their own risk assessment and actions.
- The granite on Sub Dome and Half Dome is dangerously slippery during and after rain. The cables become *much* more difficult to ascend and descend.
- Exposure to lightning increases once you are on the exposed granite above the base of Sub Dome.
- Lightning or wet rock can cause a fatal fall from either the cables or the Sub Dome steps.
- Time on the exposed section of trail (above the base of Sub Dome) will be at least 2–3 hours. Weather can change drastically during that time, and it is impossible for rangers out on the trail to make predictions.

☞ Deciding to proceed and turn around if the weather gets bad is not a good strategy. A dangerous descent in rain and/or lightning could be the result. The safest course of action is to not proceed past the base of Sub Dome during potential storm conditions.

Note: Almost all deaths and serious injuries on Half Dome and Sub Dome have happened when the rock was wet.

TIPS FOR USING THE CABLES

Wear sturdy footwear with good traction. The granite on the cable route has been worn down to a smooth, polished surface. Shoes with sticky rubber soles are recommended for the climb up the cables.

Some hikers prefer to use gloves. The steel cables can be cold and difficult to grip; if you use gloves, carry them back out with you.

Stay inside the cables. If someone needs to pass you, make room for them without going to the outside of the cables.

Use only one cable instead of both as you ascend and descend. Although it may be tempting to grip both cables (one in each hand), using both cables makes it difficult for hikers coming from the other direction to get by. Additionally, gripping both cables can sap your energy more quickly than using both hands on one cable.

OTHER MESSAGES

Pack it in, pack it out. Please keep the trail litter free! There are no trash receptacles anywhere along the trail.

Restroom locations Because the trails leading to Half Dome are so popular, several restroom facilities are available. A stone building with men's and women's flushing toilets is at the Vernal Fall Bridge. Wooden composting toilets are located at the top of Vernal Fall, at the intersection of the Upper Mist and John Muir trails, and in Little Yosemite Valley.

Appendix 3

Half Dome Hiking Accidents

This section is not here to discourage you from this hike but rather to document that it can be dangerous if you hike outside the envelope of safety. It is rare to hear or read of accidents on Half Dome. In fact, since 1919 very few people have fallen to their death when the cables are in their summer-season position. The Half Dome trail has an outstanding record of uneventful trips. The most common injuries are simple sprains or bone breaks—not the harrowing situations described below. Knowledge is power; use this knowledge to conduct a safe hike. Do not go up if the cables are down, if the rock is wet, or if there is thunder or lightning, and don't wear smooth-soled shoes. Only accidents along the Half Dome route at press time are listed here. No names are included. The park averages about 12 deaths per year. The definitive book for all types of traumatic accidents is *Off the Wall: Death in Yosemite* by Michael P. Ghiglieri and Charles R. "Butch" Farabee Jr.

Man falls off Half Dome (*August 23, 2011*) Climbers near the base of Half Dome reported seeing a man drop down the 2,000-foot face. A male body was found in the talus slopes on the Mirror Lake side of Half Dome known as the Death Slabs.

Teen dies from fall on Mist Trail (*August 9, 2011*) A 17-year-old male died from head injuries after falling on the Mist Trail.

Woman falls off Half Dome cables (*July 31, 2011*) A 26-year-old woman slipped and fell 600 feet while descending the Half Dome cables. The rock was wet from a morning rain.

Three people go over Vernal Fall (*July 19, 2011*) Ten hikers climbed over the guard railing at the top of Vernal Fall. A 21-year-old woman and 22- and 27-year-old males fell into the river and were swept over the fall.

Man dies after slipping into Merced at Mist Trail (*May 16, 2011*) A 60-year-old male slipped off the Mist Trail and slid down a slab into the Merced River. He was swept downstream several hundred feet and died.

Man commits suicide on Half Dome (*September 19, 2009*) A man committed suicide on the top of Half Dome; he shot himself while near the Visor.

Man falls off cables and dies *(June 13, 2009)* A 40-year-old male fell to his death while hiking on Half Dome; the top was pelted with hail and a cold rain.

Woman falls off cables and lives but is seriously injured *(June 6, 2009)* A 35-year-old woman slipped while descending the Half Dome cables and slid approximately 150 feet down the east face, landing on a small ledge. Half Dome was socked in with clouds, snow flurries on the summit, and mist on the cables and Sub Dome.

Woman falls into Merced and drowns *(May 18, 2009)* A 31-year-old woman slipped into the Merced River near the Vernal Fall footbridge and drowned.

Man commits suicide off Half Dome *(July 29, 2008)* A 27-year-old man leapt to his death off of 8,842-foot Half Dome.

Man falls off Half Dome cables *(June 16, 2007)* A 37-year-old male slipped and fell off the Half Dome cables while ascending.

Man falls into Merced near Vernal Fall *(June 4, 2007)* A 27-year-old male slipped into the Merced near the Vernal Fall footbridge and drowned.

Fatal fall from Half Dome cables *(April 19, 2007)* A 43-year-old woman slipped off the Half Dome cables to her death. The cables were lying on the rock in their winter mode without stanchions, which hold up the cables.

Fatal fall off Half Dome *(November 8, 2006)* A 25-year-old woman slipped off the Half Dome cables to her death. The cables were lying on the rock in their winter mode without stanchions, which hold up the cables.

Man slides down off the cables and lives! *(October 1, 2006)* A 21-year-old male slipped off the cables during inclement weather and fell nearly 200 feet, and then stopped parallel to and about 100 feet to the right of the base of the cables. He laid on his back precariously for three hours but was rescued unhurt.

Man plunges over Vernal Fall *(July, 2005)* A 24-year-old male climbed over the protective railing at Vernal Fall and walked into the water 20 feet from the edge. He slipped and fell over the edge to his death.

Lightning strike kills two *(August, 1985)* Five hikers on Half Dome took shelter in the rock "cave" enclosure at the summit during a lightning storm. One was killed by the strike, and another was shocked and fell over the edge to his death.

Appendix 4

References and Information Sources

There is much information available on Yosemite. The Internet is an invaluable repository of data. Sources used for this book include:

PRINTED MATERIAL

Browning, Peter. *John Muir in His Own Words: A Book of Quotations.* Lafayette, CA: Great West Books, 2004.

Browning, Peter. *Yosemite Place Names.* 2nd ed. Lafayette, CA: Great West Books, 2005.

Bunnell, Lafayette H. *Discovery of the Yosemite, and the Indian War of 1851, which led to that event. . .* 4th ed. Los Angeles: G. W. Gerlicher, 1911.

Carline, Jan D., Martha J. Lentz, and Steven C. MacDonald. *Mountaineering First Aid.* 5th ed. Seattle: Mountaineers Books, 2004.

Deutsch, Rick. *Yosemite's Half Dome: A Hiking Guide.* Bloomington, IN: Xlibris, 2006.

Ditton, Richard. *Yosemite Road Guide.* 2nd ed. Berkeley, CA: Yosemite Association, 1989.

Gerdes, Marti M. *Nevada Fall Corridor: A Cultural Landscape Report.* Master's thesis, University of Oregon, 2004.

Ghiglieri, Michael P., Charles R. Farabee Jr. *Off the Wall: Death in Yosemite.* Flagstaff, AZ: Puma Press, 2007.

Gillmore, Robert. *Great Walks: Yosemite National Park.* Goffstown, NH: Great Walks, Inc., 1993.

Glazner, Allen F. and Greg M. Stock. *Geology Underfoot in Yosemite National Park.* Missoula, MT: Mountain Press, 2010.

Hutchings, James. *In the Heart of the Sierras.* Oakland, CA: Pacific Press Publishing House, 1886.

Johnston, Hank. *The Yosemite Grant 1864–1906.* Berkeley, CA: Yosemite Association, 1995.

Jones, William R. *Yosemite: The Story Behind the Scenery.* Wichenburg, AZ: KC Publications, Inc., 2002

Madgic, Bob. *Shattered Air: A True Account of Catastrophe and Courage on Yosemite's Half Dome*. Short Hills, NJ: Burford Books, 2005.

Muir, John. *My First Summer in the Sierra and Selected Essays*. New York: Library of America, 2011.

O' Connell, Nick. "Half Dome." *Outside*, June 2003.

REI product information brochures (GPS, Trekking Poles, Hiking Boots, Water Filters). 2006.

Sargent, Shirley. *Pioneers in Petticoats: Yosemite's Early Women 1856–1900*. Yosemite, CA: Flying Spur Press, 2002.

Schaffer, Jeffrey P. *Hiker's Guide to the High Sierra Yosemite: The Valley and Surrounding Uplands*. 7th ed. Berkeley, CA: Wilderness Press, 2006.

Schaffer, Jeffrey P. *Yosemite National Park: A Complete Hiker's Guide*. 5th ed. Berkeley, CA: Wilderness Press, 2006.

Schaffer, Jeffrey P. *Yosemite National Park: A Natural History Guide to Yosemite and Its Trails*. Berkeley, CA: Wilderness Press, 1999.

Swedo, Suzanne. *Hiking Yosemite National Park*. 3rd ed. Guilford, CT: Falcon Publishing, 2011.

Topographic Map of Yosemite National Park and Vicinity. Berkeley, CA: Wilderness Press, 1999.

Trails of Yosemite Valley. Yosemite Association/NPS brochure, 1987.

Yosemite Today. Tabloid of park information, events, services. National Park Service and Delaware North Company. Monthly.

Yosemite: Your Complete Guide to the Park. 24th ed. 2006–2007.

WEBSITES

adventurebuddies.net   Benefits and techniques to properly use hiking poles

hikehalfdome.com   Definitive website/blog for Half Dome information

leki.com   Leading manufacturer of trekking poles

katadyn.com   Water treatment products

nps.gov/yose   National Park Service site for Yosemite

rei.com   Outdoor gear store and resource cooperative

seeyosemite.com   Commercial site with info about the park

sierraclub.org   Sierra Club website

wildernesspress.com   Comprehensive, accurate, and readable outdoor books

yosemite.ca.us/library   Scanned historical books

yosemitefun.com   Commercial, informative Yosemite info

yosemitegold.com   Commercial information for Yosemite and the Gold Country

yosemite.national-park.com   Commercial Yosemite National Park information page

yosemiteconservancy.org   Yosemite Conservancy

yosemitepark.com   DNC Parks & Resorts at Yosemite, Inc.

PHONE NUMBERS

(801) 559-5000   Lodging reservations

(209) 372-0200   Main Yosemite number; information and road conditions

(800) 436-7275   NPS campground reservations for domestic callers

(301) 722-1257   NPS campground reservations for international callers

(209) 372-0322   Save-a-Bear hotline

(800) 469-7275   Yosemite Conservancy

(209) 372-8344   Yosemite Mountaineering School

(209) 372-0740   Yosemite Wilderness Permits

VIDEOS

"#117, Half Dome." *California's Gold.* VHS. Los Angeles: Huell Howser Productions, 2002.

Else, Jon. *Yosemite: the Fate of Heaven.* VHS. Los Angeles: Sundance Institute and Yosemite Association, 1989.

Hiking Yosemite. VHS. Seattle: A. Sabo Productions, 1993.

Johnson, Sterling. *Yosemite: The 100 Year Flood: Movement in Tides.* VHS. Yosemite, CA: Yosemite Concession Services Co., 1997.

McConnell, Doug. "Half Dome." *Bay Area Backroads,* KRON.

Paley, Jayah Faye and Thomas Wohlmut. *Poles for Hiking, Trekking &Walking.* DVD. Pacifica, CA: AdventureBuddies, 2007.

Shannon, Jonathan. *Jon's DVD Hiking Guides: Yosemite National Park.* DVD. Mokelumne Hill, CA: Sierra Nomad Photography, 2010.

Vassar, David. *Spirit of Yosemite.* DVD. Berkeley, CA: The Yosemite Fund/Yosemite Association, 2002.

About the Author

Rick Deutsch lives in San Jose, California, with his wife, Diane. A veteran of Silicon Valley high tech, Rick is an adventure traveler. Some of his personal bests include rafting through the Grand Canyon (three times); ascending California's Mount Whitney and Mount Shasta; pedaling the 500-mile Iowa RAGBRAI cross-state bike tour (two times); mountain biking in Moab, Utah; 250 scuba dives, including Papua New Guinea, Palau, Truk Lagoon, the Caribbean, and the Galapagos; hiking Peru's Machu Picchu; and dogsledding in Alaska. It was after his 17th trek up Half Dome that he decided to write this guide to help others enjoy this fun and rewarding hike. As of press time, he has hiked Half Dome 31 times.

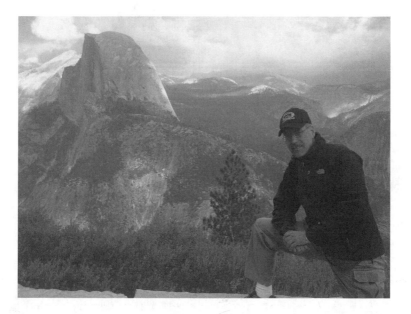

Index

More Yosemite Titles from Wilderness Press

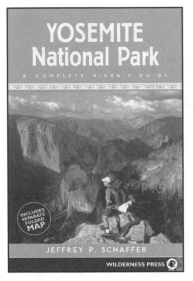
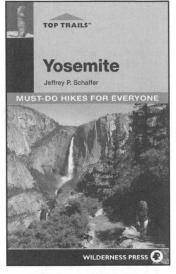
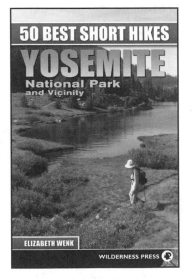